# The Story of a D

# Telephone Told by ᴛʜᴇ ᴡɪʀᴇ

Ellen M. Firebaugh

**Alpha Editions**

This edition published in 2024

ISBN : 9789362920126

Design and Setting By
**Alpha Editions**
www.alphaedis.com
Email - info@alphaedis.com

# Contents

# TO THE READER.

The telephone has revolutionized the doctor's life.

In the old days when a horse's galloping hoofs were heard people looked out of their windows and wondered if that wasn't someone after a doctor! The steed that Franklin harnessed bears the message now, and comments and curiosity are stilled. In the old days thunderous knocks came often to the doctor's door at night; they are never heard now, or so rarely as to need no mention. Neighbors have been awakened by these importunate raps: they sleep on undisturbed now.

The doctor's household enjoys nothing of this sweet immunity. A disturbing factor is within it that makes the thunderous knocks of old pale into insignificance.

When the telephone first came into the town where our doctor lived he had one put in his office of course, for if anyone in the world needs a 'phone it is the doctor and the people who want him. By and by he bethought him that since his office was several blocks from his residence he had better put one in there, too, because of calls that come in the night. So it was promptly installed. The doctor and his wife found their sleep disturbed far oftener than before. People will not dress and go out into the night to the doctor's house unless it is necessary. But it is an easy thing to step to the 'phone and call him from his sleep to answer questions—often needless—and when several people do the same thing in the same night, as frequently happens, it is not hard to see what the effect may be.

One day the doctor had an idea! He would connect the two 'phones. It would be a handy thing for Mary to be able to talk to him about the numberless little things that come up in a household without the trouble of ringing central every time, and it would be a handy thing for him, too. When he had to leave the office he could just 'phone Mary and she could keep an ear on the 'phone till he got back.

About this time another telephone system was established in the town—the Farmers'. Now a doctor's clientele includes many farmers, so he put one of the new 'phones into his office. By and by he reflected that farmers are apt to need to consult a physician at night—he must put in a Farmers' 'phone at home, too. And he did. Then he connected it with the office.

When the first 'phone went up Mary soon accustomed herself to its call— three rings. When her husband connected it with the office the rings were multiplied by three. One ring meant someone at the office calling central. Two rings meant someone calling the office. Three rings meant someone calling the residence, as before. Mary found the three calls confusing. When the Farmers' 'phone was installed and the same order of rings set up, she found the original ring multiplied by six. This was confusion worse confounded. To be sure the bell on the Farmers' had a somewhat hoarser sound than that on the Citizens' 'phone, but Mary's ear was the only one in the household that could tell the difference with certainty. The clock in the same room struck the half hours which did not tend to simplify matters. When a new door-bell was put on the front door Mary found she had eight different rings to contend with. But it is the bells of the Telephone with which we are concerned and something of their story will unfold as we proceed.

When the doctor was at home and the 'phone would ring he would start toward the adjoining room where the two hung and stop at the first.

Mary would call "Farmers'!" and he would move on to the next. Perhaps at the same instant the tall boy of the household whose ear was no more accurate than that of his father would shout "Citizens'!" and the doctor would stop between the two.

"*Farmers'!*" the wife would call a second time, with accrued emphasis. Then she would laugh heartily and declare:

"Any one coming in might think this a sort of forum where orations were being delivered," and sometimes she would go on and declaim:

"Friends, Romans, countrymen, lend me your ears—my husband has borrowed mine."

So the telephone in the doctor's house—so great a necessity that we cannot conceive of life without it, so great a blessing that we are hourly grateful for it, is yet a very great tyrant whose dominion is absolute.

I had a pleasing picture in my mind in the writing of this chronicle, of sitting serene and undisturbed in a cosy den upstairs, with all the doors between me and the 'phone shut tight where no sound might intrude. In vain. Without climbing to the attic I could not get so far away that the tintinnabulation that so mercilessly wells from those bells, bells, bells did not penetrate.

I hope my readers have not got so far away from their Poe as to imagine that ringing sentence to be mine. And I wonder if a still greater glory might not crown his brow if there had been telephone bells to celebrate in Poe's day.

So I gave up the pleasant dream, abandoned the cosy den and came down stairs to the dining room where I can scatter my manuscript about on the big table, and look the tyrants in the face and answer the queries that arise, and can sandwich in a good many little odd jobs besides.

Through a doctor's telephone how many glimpses of human nature and how many peeps into the great Story of Life have been mine; and if, while the reader is peeping too, the scene suddenly closes, why that is the way of telephones and not the fault of the writer.

And knowing how restful a thing it has been to me to get away from the ringing of the bell at times, I have devised a rest for the reader also and have sent him with the doctor and his wife on an occasional country drive where no telephone intrudes.

E. M. F.

Robinson, Ill.

The Story of a Doctor's Telephone

# CHAPTER I.

The hands of the clock were climbing around toward eleven and the doctor had not returned. Mary, a drowsiness beginning to steal over her, looked up with a yawn. Then she fell into a soliloquy:

To bed, or not to bed—that is the question:

Whether 'tis wiser in the wife to wait for a belated spouse,

Or to wrap the drapery of her couch about her

And lie down to pleasant dreams?

To dream! perchance to sleep!

And by that sleep to end the headache

And the thousand other ills that flesh is heir to,

The restoration of a wilted frame,—

Wilted by loss of sleep on previous nights—

A consummation devoutly to be wished.

To dream! perchance to sleep!—aye, there's the rub;

For in that somnolence what peals may come

Must give her pause. There is the telephone

That makes calamity of her repose.

Her spouse may not have come to answer it,

Which means that she, his wife, must issue forth

All dazed and breathless from delicious sleep,

And knock her knees on intervening chairs,

And bump her head on a half open door,

And get there finally all out of breath,

And take the receiver down and say: "Hello?"

The old, old question: "Is the doctor there?"

Comes clearly now to her awakened ear.

Then, tentatively, she must make reply:

"The doctor was called out an hour ago,

But I expect him now at any time."

Good patrons should be held and not escape

To other doctors that may lie in wait;

For in this voice so brusque and straight and clear

She recognizes an old friend and true,

Whose purse is ever ready to make good,

And she hath need of many, many things.

But then, again, the message of the 'phone

May be that of some stricken little child

Whose mother's voice trembles with love and fear.

Then must the listener earnestly advise:

"Don't wait for him! Get someone else to-night."

Perchance again the message may be that

Of colics dire and death so imminent

That she who listens, tho' with 'customed ear,

Shrinks back dismayed and knows not what to say,

Lacking the knowledge and profanity

Of him who, were he there, would settle quick

This much ado about much nothingness.

And so these anticipatory peals

Reverberate through fancy as she sits,

And make her rather choose to bear the ills

She has than fly to others she may meet;

To wait a little longer for her spouse,

That, when at last she does retire to rest,

She may be somewhat surer of her sleep.

And so she sits there waiting for the step
And the accompanying clearing of the throat
Which she would know were she in Zanzibar.
And by-and-by he comes and fate is kind
And lets them slumber till the early dawn.

# CHAPTER II.

Ten P.M. The 'phone is ringing and the sleepy doctor gets out of bed and goes to answer it.

"Hello."

No response.

"Hello!"

Silence.

"Hello!!"

"Is this Doctor Blank?"

"Yes."

"I want you to come out to my house—my wife's sick."

"Who is it?"

"Jim Warner. Come just as—"

A click in the receiver.

The doctor waits a minute. Then he says "Hello." No answer. He waits another minute. "*Hell-o!*"

Silence. "Damn that girl—she's cut us off." He hangs up the receiver and rings the bell sharply. He takes it down and hears a voice say leisurely, "D'ye get them?"

"Yes! What in h-ll did you cut us off for?"

"Wait a minute—I'll ring 'em again," says the voice, hasty and obliging, so potent a thing is a man's unveiled wrath. She rings 'em again. Soon the same voice says, "Are you there yet, Doctor?"

"Yes, *now* what is it!"

The voice proceeds and the doctor listens putting in an occasional "Yes" or "No." Then he says, "All right—I'll be out there in a little bit." He hangs up the receiver and his wife falls asleep again. The doctor dresses and goes out. The house is in darkness. All is still. In about five minutes Mary is suddenly, sharply awake. A slight noise in the adjoining room! She listens with accelerated heart-beats. The doctor has failed to put on the night latch. Some thief has been lying in wait watching for his opportunity, and now he has entered. What can she do. Muffled footsteps! she pulls the sheet over her head, her heart beating to suffocation. The footsteps grope their way toward her room! Great Heaven! A hand fumbles at the door knob. She shrieks aloud.

"What on earth is the matter!"

O, brusque and blessed is that voice!

"John, you have nearly scared me to death," she says, sitting up in bed, half laughing and half crying. "But I heard you tell that man you were coming out there."

"Yes. I told him I was."

"Well, why didn't you go?"

"I *did* go."

"You don't mean to tell me you have been a mile and back in five minutes."

The doctor flashed on the light and looked at his watch,—"Just an hour since I left home," he said. Mary gasped. "Well, it only proves how soundly I can sleep when I get a chance," she said.

Ting-a-ling-ling-ling. Ting-a-ling-ling-ling.

It is the office ring but Mary hurries at once to answer it.

"Is this Dr. Blank's office?"

"This is Mrs. Blank. But the doctor telephoned me about twenty minutes ago that he would be out for half an hour. Call him again in ten or fifteen minutes and I think you will find him."

In about fifteen minutes the call is repeated. Mary would feel better satisfied to know that the doctor received the message so she goes to the 'phone and listens. Silence. She waits a minute. Shall she speak? She hesitates. Struggle as she will against the feeling, she can't quite overcome it—it seems like "butting in." But that long silence with the listening ear at the other end of it is too much for her. Very pleasantly, almost apologetically she asks, "What is it?"

"The doctor hasn't come yet?" says a plainly disappointed voice.

"No—not yet. There are often unexpected things to delay him—if you will give me your number or your name I will have him call *you*."

"No, I'll just wait and call him again." The inflection says plainly, "I don't care to admit the doctor's wife into my confidences."

"Very well. I am sure it can't be long now till he returns."

Mary goes back to her chair and ponders a little. Of what avail to multiply words. No use to tell the woman 'phoning that she was willing to take the waiting and the watching, the seeing that the doctor received the message upon herself rather than that the other should be again troubled by it. No use to let her gently understand that she doesn't care for any confidences which belong only to her husband, but Fate has placed her in a position where she has oftentimes to seem unduly interested. That these messages which are only occasional with the one calling are constant with her and that she is only mindful of them when she must be.

"Watch the 'phone." How thoroughly instilled into Mary's consciousness that admonition was! She did not heed the office ring when it came, but if it came a second time she always went to explain that the doctor had just stepped over to the drug store probably and would be back in a very few minutes. Often, as she stood explaining, the doctor himself would break into the conversation, having been in another room when the first call came, and getting there a little tardily for the second. But occasions sometimes arose which made Mary feel very thankful that she had been at the 'phone. One winter morning as she stood explaining to some woman that the doctor would be in in a few minutes, her husband's "Hello" was heard.

"There he is now," she said. Usually after this announcement she would hang up the receiver and go about her work. Today a friendly interest in this pleasant voice kept it in her hand a moment. Mary would not have admitted idle curiosity, and perhaps she had as little of it as falls to the lot of women, but sometimes she lingered a moment for the message, to know if the doctor was to be called away, so that she might make her plans for dinner accordingly. The pleasant voice spoke again, "This is Dr. Blank, is it?"

"Yes."

"We want you to come out to Henry Ogden's."

"That's about five miles out, isn't it. Who's sick out there?"

"Mrs. Ogden."

"What's the matter?"

No reply.

"How long has she been sick?"

"She began complaining last night."

"All right—I'll be out some time today."

"Come right away, please, if you can."

This is an old, old plea. The doctor is thoroughly inured to it. He would have to be twenty men instead of one to respond to it at all times. He answers cheerfully, "All right," and Mary takes alarm. That tone means sometime in the next few hours. She feels sure he ought to go *now*. Somebody else can wait better than this patient. There was a kind of hesitancy in that voice that Mary had heard before. A woman's intuitions are much safer guides than a man's slow reasoning. She must speak to John. She rings the office.

"Hello."

"Say, John," she says in a low voice, "I came to the 'phone thinking you were out and heard that message. I think you ought to go out there right *away*."

"Well, I'm going after a little."

"But I don't think you ought to wait. I'm sure it's—*you* know."

"Well,—maybe I had better go right out."

"I wish you would. I know they'll be looking for you every minute."

A few minutes later Mary saw him drive past and was glad. Half an hour later the office ring sounded. She did not wait for the second peal. True, John had not said, "Watch the 'phone," today, but that was understood. Occasionally he got an old man who lived next door to the office to come in and stay during his absence. Possibly he might have done so today. But even if he were there the telephone and its ways were a dark mystery to him and besides, his deafness made him of little use in that direction.

Mary took down the receiver and put it to her ear. A lady's voice was asking, "Who *is* this?"

Mary knew from her inflection that she had asked something before and was not satisfied with the reply.

"*This* is Dr. Blank's office?" announced the old man in a sort of interrogative.

"Well, where is the *doctor*?"

"The doctor," said the old man meditatively, as if wondering that anybody should be calling for him—"the doctor—you mean Dr. Blank, I reckon?"

"I certainly do."

"Good Heavens," thought Mary, "why *don't* he go on!"

"Why, he's out."

"Where *is* he?"

"He went to the country."

Mary shut her lips tight.

"*Well*, when will he be back?"

"He 'lowed he'd be back in about an hour or so."

"How long has he been *gone*? Maybe I'll get some information after a while."

Mary longed to speak. Why hadn't she done so at first. If she thrust herself in now it would make her out an eavesdropper. But this was unbearable. She opened her mouth to speak when the old man answered.

"He's been gone over an hour now, I reckon."

"Then he'll soon be back. Will you be there when he comes?"

"Yes ma'am."

"Then tell him to come up to Mrs. Dorlan's."

"To Mrs. Who's?"

"Mrs. *Dorlan's*."

"I didn't ketch the name."

"*Mrs. Dorlan's*, on Brownson street."

"Mrs. Torren's?"

"MISS-ES—DOR-LAN'S!" shouted the voice.

Mary sighed fiercely and clinched her teeth unconsciously. "I *will* speak," she thought, when the old voice ventured doubtingly,

"Mrs. Dorlan's?"

"That's it. Mrs. Dorlan's on Brownson street, will you remember it?"

"Mrs. Dorlan's, on Brownson street."

"That's right. Please tell him just as soon as he comes to come right up."

"All right—I'll tell him."

"Poor old fellow!" said Mary as she turned from the 'phone, "but I don't want to go through any more ordeals like that. It was a good deal harder for me than for the other woman."

The doctor came down late to dinner. "You got Mrs. Dorlan's message did you?"

"Yes, I'll go up there right after dinner." He looked at his wife with peculiar admiration.

"How did you know what was wanted with me out in the country?" he asked.

With a little pardonable pride she replied: "Oh, I just felt it. Women have ways of understanding each other that men never attain to. Is it a boy or a girl added to the world today?"

"Neither," said the doctor placidly, helping himself to a roll.

Chagrin overspread her face. "Well," she said with an embarrassed smile, "I erred on mercy's side, and it *might* have happened in just that way, John, and you know it."

The doctor laughed. "There was mighty little the matter out there—they didn't need a doctor."

"Are they good pay?"

"Good as old wheat."

"Then there are compensations."

Some hours later when the 'phone rang, Mary went to explain that the doctor had 'phoned her he would be out about twenty minutes. But she found no chance to speak. A spirited dialogue was taking place between a young man and a maid:

"Where *are* you, Jack?"

"I'm right here."

"Smarty! Where *are* you!"

"In Dr. Blank's office."

"What are you there for?"

"I'm waiting for the doctor and to while away the time thought I'd call you up."

Then it was his ring that Mary had answered. "I ought to hang this receiver right up," thought she, but instead she held it, her face beaming with a sympathetic smile.

"Are you feeling better today, Dolly?"

"Yes, I'm better."

"Able to go to the show then, tonight?"

"*Yes*, I'm able to go."

Here a thin small voice put in, "No, you're not able! You're not going."

"Mamma says,—" began a pouting voice.

"I heard what she said," said Jack, laughing. "Have you been up all day?"

"Most of the day."

"Can you eat anything?"

"I ate an egg, some toast and some fruit for dinner."

"That's fine. I'll bring you a box of candy then pretty soon—I'm coming down in a little bit."

"That will be lovely."

"Which, the candy or the coming down?"

"The candy, goose, of course." A laugh at both ends of the wire.

Then Jack's voice. "Well, here comes the doctor. I've got to have my neck amputated now. Goodbye."

"Good-bye."

"All's fair in love and war," said Mary, "and it's plain to see what this is." Then she hung up the receiver without a qualm.

There were other times when the doctor's wife was glad she had gone to the 'phone, as in this instance.

She had taken down the receiver when a man's voice said, "The doctor just stepped out for a few minutes. If you will tell me your name, madam, I'll have him call you when he comes in."

Disinterested courtesy spoke in his voice, but Mary was not in the least surprised to hear the curt reply, "It won't be necessary. I'll call *him* when he comes."

"I dare say that gentleman, whoever he may be, is wondering what he has done," thought Mary.

But it was not altogether unpleasant to her to hear somebody else squelched, too!

There came a day when the doctor's wife rebelled. When her husband came home and ate his supper hastily and then rose to depart, she said, "You'd better wait at home a few minutes, John."

"Why?" He put the question brusquely, his hat in his hand.

"Because I think someone will ring here for you in a minute or two. Some man rang the office twice so I went to the 'phone to explain that you must be on your way to supper and he could find you here."

"Who was it?"

"I do not know."

"Thunder! Why didn't you find out?"

Mary looked straight at her husband. "How many times have I told you, John, that many people decline to give their names or their messages to any one but you. I think I should feel that way about it myself. For a long time I have dutifully done your bidding in the matter, but now I vow I will not trample my pride under my feet any longer—especially when it is all in vain. I will watch the 'phone as faithfully as in the past, but I will not ask for any name or any message. They will be given voluntarily if at all."

"All right, Mary," said the doctor, gently, seeing that she was quite serious.

"I do not mean to say that most of the people who 'phone are grouchy and disagreeable—far from it. Indeed the majority are pleasant and courteous. But it is those who are not who have routed me, and made me vow my vow. Don't ask me to break it, John, for I will not."

And having delivered this declaration, Mary felt almost as free and independent as in ante-telephone days.

The doctor had seated himself and leaning forward was swinging his hat restlessly between his knees. He waited five minutes.

"I'll have to get back to the office," he exclaimed, starting up. "I'm expecting a man to pay me some money. Waiting for the 'phone to ring is like watching for the pot to boil."

When he had been gone a minute or two, the ring came. With a new step Mary advanced to it.

"Has the doctor got there yet?" the voice had lost none of its grouch.

"He has. And he waited for your message which did not come. He could not wait longer. He has just gone to the office. If you will 'phone him there in two or three minutes, instead of waiting till he is called out again, you will find him."

"Thank you, Mrs. Blank." The man was surprised into courtesy.

The clear-cut, distinct sentences were very different from the faltering, apologetic ones, when she had asked for his name or his message twenty minutes before.

Mary's receiver clicked with no uncertain sound and a smile illumined her face.

One day when the snow was flying and the wind was blowing a gale the doctor came hurrying in. "Where is the soapstone?" he asked, with small amenity. His wife flew to get it and laid it on the hearth very close to the coals. "Oh dear! How terrible to go out in such a storm. Do you *have* to?" she asked.

"I certainly do. Do you think I'd choose a day like this for a pleasure trip?"

"Aren't you glad you got that galloway?" she asked, hurrying to bring the big, hairy garment from its hook in the closet. She helped her husband into it, turned the broad collar up—then, when the soapstone was hot, she wrapped it up and gave it to him. "This ought to keep your feet from freezing," she said. The doctor took it, hurried out to the buggy, pulled the robes up around him and was gone.

"Eight miles in this blizzard!" thought Mary shivering, "and eight miles back—sixteen miles. It will take most of the day."

Two hours after the doctor had gone the telephone rang.

"Is Dr. Blank there?"

"No, he is in the country, about eight miles southwest."

"This is Drayton. We want him at John Small's as soon as possible. How soon do you think he will be back?"

"Not for several hours, I am afraid."

"Well, will you send him down as soon as he comes? We want him *bad*."

Mary assured him she would do so. "Poor John," she thought as she put up the receiver.

In a few minutes she went hurriedly back. When she had called central, she said, "I am very anxious to get Dr. Blank, central. He is eight miles southwest of here—at the home of Thomas Calhoun. Is there a 'phone there?" Silence for a few seconds then a voice, "No, there is no 'phone at Thomas Calhoun's."

Disappointed, Mary stood irresolute, thinking. Then she asked,

"Is there a 'phone at Mr. William Huntley's?"

"Yes, William Huntley has a 'phone."

"Thank you. Please call that house for me."

In a minute a man's voice said, "Hello."

"Is this Mr. Huntley?"

"Yes."

"Mr. Huntley, this is Mrs. Blank. You live not far from Thomas Calhoun's, do you not?"

"About half a mile."

"Dr. Blank is there, or will be very soon, and there is an urgent call for him to go on to Drayton. I want to save him the long drive home first. I find there is no 'phone at Mr. Calhoun's so I have called you hoping you might be able to help me out. Perhaps someone of your family will be going down that way and will stop in."

"I'll go, myself."

"It's too bad to ask any one to go out on a day like this—"

"That's all right, Mrs. Blank. Doc's been pretty clever to me."

"Tell him, please, to go to John Small's at Drayton. I am very deeply obliged to you for your kindness, Mr. Huntley," she said, hanging the receiver in its place.

"Eight miles back home, six miles from here to Drayton, six miles back— twenty miles in all. Four miles from Calhoun's to Drayton, six miles from Drayton home—ten miles saved on a blizzardy day," she thought in the thankfulness of her heart.

A few minutes later she was again at the 'phone. "Please give me John Small's at Drayton." When the voice came she said, "I wanted to tell you that the doctor will be there perhaps in about an hour now. I got your message to him so that he will go directly to your house."

"I'm mighty glad to know it. Thank you, Mrs. Blank, for finding him and for letting us know."

A terrible drive saved and some anxious hearts relieved. That dear 'phone! How thankful she was for it and for the country drives she had taken with her husband which had made her familiar with the homes and names of many farmers. Otherwise she could not have located her husband this morning. One day like this covered a multitude of tyrannies from the little instrument on the wall.

It was about half past seven. The doctor had thought it probable that he could get off early this evening and then he and Mary and the boys would have a game of whist. He had been called in consultation to W., a little town in an adjoining county, but he would be home in a little bit—in just ten minutes the train would be due.

"O, there goes that 'phone," said the small boy wrathfully. "Now, I s'pose papa can't get here!"

His mother was already there with the receiver at her ear.

"This is Dr. Blank's residence."

"No, but he will be here in fifteen or twenty minutes."

"To Drayton?"

"Very well. I will give him your message as soon as he gets home. I'm afraid that ends the game for tonight, boys," putting the receiver up.

"Why, does papa have to go away?"

"Yes, he has to drive six miles."

"Gee-mi-nee—this dark night in the mud!"

Here a thought flashed into Mary's mind—Drayton was on the same railroad on which the doctor was rapidly nearing home—the next station beyond. She flew to the telephone and rang with nervous haste.

"Hello."

"Is this the Big Four?"

"Yes."

"This is Mrs. Blank. Dr. Blank is on the train which is due now. He is wanted at Drayton. When he gets off, will you please tell him?"

"To go on to Drayton?"

"Yes, to Alfred Walton's."

"All right. I'll watch for him and see that he gets aboard again."

"Thank you very much."

The train whistled. "Just in time," said Mary.

"But how'll papa get back?" asked the smaller boy.

"He's got a tie-ticket," said his brother.

"Yes, papa would rather walk back on the railroad than drive both ways through this deep mud," said their mother. "I have heard him say so."

Another ring.

"Is the doctor there?"

"He has just gone on the train to Drayton."

"How soon will he be back?"

"In an hour and a half, I should think."

Mary heard the 'phoner say in an aside, "He won't be back for an hour and a half. Do you want to wait that long?"

Another voice replied, "Yes, I'll wait. Tell 'em to tell him to come just as quick as he gets back, though."

This message was transmitted.

"And where is he to go?"

"To Henry Smith's, down by the Big Four depot."

A few minutes later Mary had another idea. She went to the 'phone and asked central to give her Drayton, Mr. Walton's house.

In a minute a voice said, "What is it?" It was restful to Mary to have the usual opening varied. Perhaps eight out of ten began with,

"Hello!" The other two began, "Yes," "Well," "What is it?" and very rarely, "Good morning," or "Good evening."

"Is this the home of Mr. Walton at Drayton?"

"Yes."

"Dr. Blank is there just now, isn't he?"

"Yes, but he's just going away."

"Will you please ask him to come to the 'phone?"

In a minute her husband's voice was heard asking what was wanted.

"I want to save you a long walk when you get home, John. You're wanted at Henry Smith's down by the Big Four depot."

"All right. I'll go in to see him when I get there. Much obliged."

"A mile walk saved there," mused the doctor's wife, as she joined the two boys, mildly grumbling because they couldn't have their game, and never could have it just when they wanted it. But a few chapters from Ivanhoe read to them by their mother made all serene again.

The Citizens' 'phone was ringing persistently. The doctor's wife had been upstairs and could not get to it in less than no time! But she got there.

"Do you know where Dr. Blank is?" the words hurled themselves against her ear.

"I don't know just at this minute—but he's here in town. I'm sure of that."

"Why don't he *come* then!" The sentence came as from a catapult.

"I don't know anything about it. Where was he to go?"

A scornful "*Huh!*" came over the wire—"I guess you forgot to tell 'im."

"I have not been asked to tell him anything this morning."

There was heated silence for an instant, then a voice big with wrath:

"You told me not fifteen minutes ago that you would send him right down."

"You are mistaken," said Mary gently but firmly. "This is the first time I have been at the 'phone this morning."

"Well, what do you think of that!" This was addressed to someone at the other end of the line, but it came clearly to Mary's ear and its intonation said volumes.

"You're the very identical woman that told me when I 'phoned awhile ago that you'd send him right down. It's the very same voice."

"There is a mistake somewhere," reiterated Mary, patiently, "but I'll send the doctor as soon as he gets in if you will give me your name."

"I'll tell ye agin, then, that he's to come to Lige Thornton's."

"Very well. I'll send him," and Mary left the 'phone much mystified. "She was in dead earnest—and so was I. I can't understand it." Glancing out of the window she saw her tall, young daughter coming up the walk. The solution came with lightning quickness—strange she didn't think of that, Gertrude had answered. She remembered now that others had thought their voices very much alike, especially over the 'phone. "If the woman had not talked in such a cyclonic way I would have thought of it," she reflected.

When the young girl entered the room her mother said, "Gertrude, you answered the 'phone awhile ago, didn't you?"

"About twenty minutes ago. Some woman was so anxious for father to come right away that I just ran down to the office to see that he *went*."

"That was very thoughtful of you, dear, but it's little credit we're getting for it."

She related the dialogue that had just taken place and mother and daughter laughed in sympathy.

"Why, Mamma, we couldn't forget if we wanted to. That telephone is an Old Man of the Sea to both of us—is now and ever shall be, world without end."

"But did you find your father at the office?"

"Yes, and waited till he fixed up some medicine for two patients already waiting, then shooed him out before some more came in. I wanted to get it off *my* mind."

"I'm glad he is on his way. Now stay within hearing of the 'phone, dearie, till I finish my work up-stairs."

"All right, Mamma, I'm going to make a cake now, but I can hear the 'phone plainly from the kitchen."

It wasn't long till a ring was heard. Gertrude dusted the flour from her hands and started. "Which 'phone was it?" she asked the maid.

"I think it was the Farmers'," said Mollie, hesitating.

So to the Farmers' 'phone went Gertrude.

"Hello."

No answer.

"Hello."

Silence.

She clapped the receiver up and hurried to the Citizens' 'phone.

"Hello."

"Is this Dr. Blank's?"

"Yes."

"Is he there?"

"No, he was called—" Here a loud ring from the other 'phone sounded.

"He was called down to—" said Gertrude rapidly, then paused, unable to think of the name at the instant.

"If you will tell me where he went, I'll just 'phone down there for him," said the voice.

A second peal from the other 'phone.

"*Yes, yes!*" said Gertrude impatiently. "O, I didn't mean that for you," she hurried apologetically. "The other 'phone is calling, and I'm so confused I can't think. Will you excuse me just an instant till I see what is wanted?"

"Certainly."

She flew to the Farmers' 'phone.

"Is this Dr. Blank's?"

"Yes."

"Good while a-answerin'," grumbled a voice.

"I did answer but no one answered *me*."

"Where's the doctor?"

"He's down in the east part of town—will be back in a little bit."

"Well, when he comes tell him—just hold the 'phone a minute, will you, till I speak to my wife."

"All right." But she put the receiver swiftly up and rushed back to the waiting man. She could answer him and get back by the time the other was ready for her.

"Hello, still there?"

"Yes."

"I've thought of the name—father went to Elijah Thornton's."

"Thornton's—let's see—have you a telephone directory handy—could you give me their number?"

"Wait a minute, I'll see." She raced through the pages,—"yes, here it is."

A violent peal from the Farmers' 'phone. "He'll think I'm still hunting for the number," she thought, letting the receiver hang and rushing to the other 'phone.

"Hello."

"Thought you was a-goin' to hold the 'phone. I've had a turrible time gittin' any answer."

"I've had a turrible time, too," thought poor Gertrude.

"Tell the doctor to call me up," and he gave his name and his number.

"All right, I'll tell him." She clapped the receiver up lest there might be more to follow and sped back.

"Here it is," she announced calmly, "Elijah Thornton, number 101."

"Thank you, I'm afraid I've put you to a good deal of trouble."

"Not at all."

As she went back to her cake she said to herself, "Two telephones ringing at once can certainly make things interesting."

One day in mid winter Mary sat half dreaming before the glowing coals. Snow had fallen all through the previous night and today there had been good coasting for the boys and girls.

Ting-a-ling-ling-ling. Ting-a-ling-ling-ling. Ting-a-ling-ling-ling.

She started up and went to answer it.

"Is this you, Mary?"

"Yes."

"I'll be out of the office about twenty minutes."

"Very well."

Sometimes Mary wished her husband would be a little more explicit. She had a vague sort of feeling that central, or whoever should chance to hear him make this announcement to her so often, might think she requested or perhaps demanded it; might think she wanted to know every place her husband went.

In about half an hour the 'phone rang again, two rings.

John ought to be back. Should she take it for granted? It would be safer to put the receiver to her ear and listen for her husband's voice.

"Hello."

"Hello."

"Is this you Dr. Blank?"

"Looks like it."

"We want ye to come down to our house right away."

"Who is this?"

"W'y, this is Mrs. Peters."

"Mrs. Peters? Oh yes," said the doctor, recognizing the voice now.

"What's the matter down there, grandmother?"

"W'y—my little grandson, Johnny, was slidin' down hill on a board and got a splinter in his setter."

"He did, eh?"

"Yes, he did, and a big one, too."

"Well, I'll be down there right away. Have some boiled water."

Mary turned away from the telephone that it might not register her low laughter as she put the receiver in its place. The next instant she took it down again with twinkling eyes and listened. Yes, the voices were silent, it would be safe. She rang two rings.

"Hello," said her husband's voice.

"John," said Mary, almost in a whisper, "for English free and unadorned, commend me to a little boy's grandmother!"

Two laughs met over the wire, then two receivers clicked.

One day Mary came in from a walk and noticed at once, a vacant place on the wall where the Farmers' 'phone had hung. She had heard rumors of a merger of the two systems and had fervently hoped that they might merge soon and forever.

"Look! Mamma," said Gertrude, pointing to the wall.

"Oh frabjous day! Callooh! Callay!

One telephone is taken away!"

she chortled in her joy.

(The small boy of the household had been reading "Alice" and consequently declaiming the Jabberwock from morning till night, till its weird strains had become fixed in the various minds of the household and notably in Gertrude's.)

"It will simplify matters," said her mother, smiling, "but liberty is not for us. *That* tuneful peal will still ring on," and as she looked at the Citizens' 'phone the peal came.

# CHAPTER III.

One Monday evening the doctor and his wife sat chatting cosily before the fire. In the midst of their conversation, Mary looked up suddenly. "I had a queer little experience this morning, John, I want to tell you about it."

"Tell ahead," said John, propping his slippered feet up on the fender.

"Well, I got my pen and paper ready to write a letter to Mrs. E. I wanted to write it yesterday afternoon and tell her some little household incidents just while they were taking place, as she is fond of the doings and sayings of boys and they are more realistic if reported in the present tense. But I couldn't get at it yesterday afternoon. When I started to write it this morning it occurred to me to date the letter Sunday afternoon and write it just as I would have done yesterday—so I did. When I had got it half done or more I heard the door-bell and going to open it I saw through the large glass—"

Ting-a-ling-ling-ling. Ting-a-ling-ling-ling.

The doctor went to the 'phone.

"Yes."

"Yes."

"Where do you live?"

"I'll be right down."

He went back, hastily removed his slippers and began putting on his shoes. Mary saw that he had clean forgotten her story. Very well. It wouldn't take more than a minute to finish it—there would be plenty of time while he was getting into his shoes—but if he was not enough interested to refer to it again she certainly would not. In a few minutes the doctor was gone and Mary went to bed. An hour or two later his voice broke in upon her slumber. "Back again," he said as he settled down upon his pillow. In a minute he exclaimed, "Say, Mary, what was the rest of that story?"

"O, don't get me roused up. I'm *so* sleepy," she said drowsily.

"Well, I'd like to hear it." The interest in her little story which had not been exhibited at the proper time was being exhibited now with a vengeance. She sighed and said, "I can't think of it now—tell you in the morning. Good night," and turned away.

When morning came and they were both awake, the doctor again referred to the unfinished story.

"It's lost interest for me. It wasn't a story to start with, just a little incident that seemed odd—"

"Well, let's have it."

"Well, then," said Mary, "I was writing away when the door-bell rang. I went to open it and saw through the glass the laundry man—"

Ting-a-ling-ling-ling. Ting-a-ling-ling-ling. Ting-a-ling-ling-ling.

"Go on!" exclaimed her husband, hurriedly, "I'll wait till you finish."

"I'll not *race* through a story in any such John Gilpin style," said Mary, tartly. "Go, John!"

The doctor arose and went.

"No."

"I think not."

"Has she any fever?"

"All right, I'll be down in a little bit."

Then he went back. "Now you can finish," he said.

"Finis is written *here*," said Mary. "Don't say story to me again!" So Mary's story remained unfinished.

But a few days later, when she was in the buggy with her husband she relented. "Now that the 'phone can't cut me short, John, I will finish about the odd incident just because you wanted to know. But it will fall pretty flat now, as all things do with too many preliminary flourishes."

"Go on," said the doctor.

"Well, you know I told you I dated my letter back to Sunday afternoon, and was writing away when I heard the door-bell ring. As I started toward the door I saw the laundry man standing there. I was conscious of looking at him in astonishment and in a dazed sort of way as I walked across the large room to open the door. I am sure he must have noticed the expression on my face. When I opened the door he asked as he always does, 'Any laundry?'"

"'Any laundry *today*?' The words were on my tongue's end but I stopped them in time. You see it was really Sunday to me, so deep into the spirit of it had I got, and it was with a little shock that I came back to Monday again in time to answer the man in a rational way. And now my story's done."

"Not a bad one, either," said John, "I'm glad you condescended to finish it."

The doctor came home at ten o'clock and went straight to bed and to sleep. At eleven he was called.

"What is it?" he asked gruffly.

"It's time for Silas to take his medicine and he won't do it."

"Won't, eh?"

"No, he vows he won't."

"Well, let him alone for a while and then try again."

About one came another ring.

"We've both been asleep, Doctor, but I've been up fifteen minutes trying to get him to take his medicine and he won't do it. He says it's too damned nasty and that he don't need it anyhow."

"Tell him I say he's a mighty good farmer, but a devilish poor doctor."

"I don't know what to do. I can't make him take it."

"You'll have to let him alone for awhile I guess, maybe he'll change his mind after awhile."

At three o'clock the doctor was again at the telephone.

"Doctor, he just will *not* take it," the voice was now quite distressed. "I can't manage him at all."

"You *ought* to manage him. What's a wife for? Well, go to bed and don't bother him or me any more tonight."

But early next morning Silas' wife telephoned again.

"I thought I ought to tell you that he hasn't taken it yet."

"He'll get well anyway. Don't be a bit uneasy about *him*," said the doctor, laughing, as he rung off.

"It's time to go, John."

Mary was drawing on her gloves. She looked at her moveless husband as he sat before the crackling blaze in the big fireplace.

"This is better than church," he made reply.

"But you promised you would go tonight. Come on."

"It isn't time yet, is it?"

"The last bell will ring before we get there."

"Well, let's wait till all that singing's over. That just about breaks my back."

Mary sat down resignedly. If they missed the singing perhaps John would not look at his watch and sigh so loud during the sermon. And it might not be a bad idea to miss the singing for another reason. The last time John had gone to church he had astonished her by sliding up beside her, taking hold of the hymn-book and singing! It happened to be his old favorite, "Sweet fields beyond the swelling flood."

Of course it was lovely that he should want to sing it with her—but the *way* he sang it! He was in the wrong key and he came out two or three syllables behind on most of the lines, but undismayed by the sudden curtailment went boldly ahead on the next. And Mary had been much relieved when the hymn was ended and the book was closed. So now she waited very patiently for her husband to make some move toward starting. By and by he got up and they went out. No sooner was the door closed behind them than the "ting-a-ling-ling-ling" was heard. The doctor threw open the door and went back. Mary, waiting at the threshold, heard one side of the dialogue.

"Yes."

"Down where?"

"Shake up your 'phone. I can't hear you."

"That's better. Now what is it?"

"Swallowed benzine, did she? How much?... That won't kill her. Give her some warm water to drink. And give her a spoonful of mustard—anything to produce vomiting...... She has? That's all right. Tell her to put her finger down her throat and vomit some more..... No, I think it won't be necessary for me to come down..... You would? Well, let me hear again in the next hour or two, and if you still want me I'll come. Good-bye."

They walked down the street and as they drew near the office they saw the figure of the office boy in the doorway silhouetted against the light within. He was looking anxiously in their direction. Suddenly he disappeared and the faint sound of a bell came to their ears. They quickened their pace and as they came up the boy came hurriedly to the door again.

"Is that you, Doctor?" he asked, peering out.

"Yes."

"I told a lady at the 'phone to wait a minute, she's 'phoned twice." Mary waited at the door while her husband went into the office and over to the 'phone.

"Yes. What is it?.... No. No. *No!*.... Listen to me..... Be *still* and listen to *me!* She's in no more danger of dying than *you* are. She couldn't die if she tried..... Be still, I say, and listen to me!" He stamped his foot mightily. Mary laughed softly to herself. "Now don't hang over her and *sympathize* with her; that's exactly what she don't need. And don't let the neighbors hang around her either. Shut the whole tea-party out..... Well, tell 'em *I* said so..... I don't care a damn *what* they think. Your duty and mine is to do the very best we can for that girl. Now remember..... Yes, I'll be down on the nine o'clock train tomorrow morning. Good-bye." He joined his wife at the door. "If anybody wants me, come to the church," he said, turning to the boy.

Mary laid her hand within her husband's arm and they started on. They met a man who stopped and asked the doctor how soon he would be at the office, as he was on his way there to get some medicine.

"I'd better go back," said the doctor and back they went. It seemed to Mary that her husband might move with more celerity in fixing up the medicine. He was deliberation itself as he cut and arranged the little squares of paper. Still more deliberately he heaped the little mounds of white powder upon them. She looked on anxiously. At last he was ready to fold them up! No, he reached for another bottle. He took out the cork, but his spatula was not in sight. Nowise disturbed, he shifted bottles and little boxes about on the table.

"Can't you use your knife, Doctor?" asked Mary.

"O, I'll find it—it's around here somewhere." In a minute or two the missing spatula was discovered under a paper, and then the doctor slowly, *so* slowly, dished out little additions to the little mounds. Then he laid the spatula up, put the cork carefully back in the bottle, turned in his chair and put two questions to the waiting man, turned back and folded the mounds in the squares with the most painstaking care. In spite of herself Mary fidgeted and when the powders with instructions were delivered and the man had gone, she rose hastily. "*Do* come now before somebody else wants something."

The singing was over and the sermon just beginning when they reached the church. It progressed satisfactorily to the end. The doctor usually made an important unit in producing that "brisk and lively air which a sermon inspires when it is quite finished." But tonight, a few minutes before the finale came, Mary saw the usher advancing down the aisle. He stopped at their seat and bending down whispered something to the doctor, who turned and whispered something to his wife.

"No, I'll stay and walk home with the Rands. I see they're here," she whispered back.

The doctor rose and went out. "Who's at the office?" he asked, as he walked away with the boy.

"She's not there yet, she telephoned. I told her you was at church."

"Did she say she couldn't wait?"

"She said she had been at church too, but a bug flew in her ear and she had to leave, and she guessed you'd have to leave too, because she couldn't stand it. She said it felt *awful*."

"Where is she?"

"She was at a house by the Methodist church, she said, when she 'phoned to see if you was at the office. When I told her I'd get you from the other church, she said she'd be at the office by the time you got there."

And she was, sitting uneasily in a big chair.

"Doctor, I've had a flea in my ear sometimes, but this is a different proposition. Ugh! Please get this creature out *now*. It feels as big as a bat. Ugh! It's crawling further in, hurry!"

"Maybe we'd better wait a minute and see if it won't be like some other things, in at one ear and out at the other."

"O, hurry, it'll get so far in you can't reach it."

"Turn more to the light," commanded the doctor, and in a few seconds he held up the offending insect.

"O, you only got a little of it!"

"I got it all."

"Well, it certainly felt a million times bigger than that," and she departed radiantly happy.

# CHAPTER IV.

One day in early spring the doctor surprised his wife by asking her if she would like to take a drive.

"In March? The roads are not passable yet, surely."

But the doctor assured her that the roads were getting pretty good except in spots. "I have such a long journey ahead of me today that I want you to ride out as far as Centerville and I can pick you up as I come back."

"That's seven or eight miles. I'll go. I can stop at Dr. Parkin's and chat with Mrs. Parkin till you come."

Accordingly a few minutes later the doctor and Mary were speeding along through the town which they soon left far behind them.

About two miles out they saw a buggy down the road ahead of them which seemed to be at a stand-still. When they drew near they found a woman at the horses' heads with a broken strap in her hand. She was gazing helplessly at the buggy which stood hub-deep in mud. She recognized the doctor and called out, "Dr. Blank, if ever I needed a doctor in my life, it's now."

"Stuck fast, eh?"

The doctor handed the reins to his wife and got out.

"I see—a broken single-tree. Well, I always unload when I get stuck, so the first thing we do we'll take this big lummox out of here," he said picking his way to the buggy. The lummox rose to her feet with a broad grin and permitted herself to be taken out. She was a fat girl about fourteen years old.

"My! I'll bet she weighs three hundred pounds," observed the doctor when she was landed, which was immediately resented. Then he took the hitching-rein and tied the tug to the broken end of the single-tree; after which he went to the horses' heads and commanded them to "Come on." They started and the next instant the vehicle was on terra firma. Mother and daughter gave the doctor warm thanks and each buggy went its separate way.

Mary was looking about her. "The elms have a faint suspicion that spring is coming; the willows only are quite sure of it," she said, noting their tender greenth which formed a soft blur of color, the only color in all the gray landscape. No, there is a swift dash of blue, for a jay has settled down on the top of a rail just at our travelers' right.

Soon they were crossing a long and high bridge spanning a creek which only a week before had been a raging torrent; the drift, caught and held by the trunks of the trees, and the weeds and grasses all bending in one direction, told the story. But the waters had subsided and now lay in deep, placid pools.

"Stop, John, quick!" commanded Mary when they were about half way across. The doctor obeyed wondering what could be the matter. He looked at his wife, who was gazing down into the pool beneath.

"I suppose I'm to stop while you count all the fish you can see."

"I was looking at that lovely concave sky down there. See those two white clouds floating so serenely across the blue far, far below the tip-tops of the elm trees."

The doctor drove relentlessly on.

"Another mudhole," said Mary after a while, "but this time the travelers tremble on the brink and fear to launch away."

When they came up they found a little girl standing by the side of the horse holding up over its back a piece of the harness. She held it in a very aimless and helpless way. "See," said Mary, "she doesn't know what to do a bit more than I should. I wonder if she can be alone."

The doctor got out and went forward to help her and discovered a young man sitting cozily in the carriage. He glanced at him contemptuously.

"Your harness is broken, have you got a string?" he asked abruptly.

"N-n-o, I haven't," said the youth feeling about his pockets.

"Take your shoe-string. If you haven't got one I'll give you mine," and he set his foot energetically on the hub of the wheel to unlace his shoe.

"Why, I've got one here, I guess," and the young man lifted a reluctant foot. The doctor saw and understood. The little sister was to fix the harness in order to save her brother's brand new shoes from the mud.

"You'd better fix that harness yourself, my friend, and fix it strong," was the doctor's parting injunction as he climbed into the buggy and started on.

"I don't like the looks of this slough of despond," said Mary. The next minute the horses were floundering through it, tugging with might and main. Now the wheels have sunk to the hubs and the horses are straining every muscle.

"Merciful heaven!" gasped Mary. At last they were safely through, and the doctor looking back said, "That is the last great blot on our civilization—bad roads."

After a while there came from across the prairie the ascending, interrogative *boo-oo-m* of a prairie chicken not far distant, while from far away came the faint notes of another. And now a different note, soft, melodious and mournful is heard.

"How far away do you think that dove is?" asked the doctor.

"It sounds as if it might be half a mile."

"It is right up here in this tree in the field."

"Is it," said Mary, looking up. "Yes, I see, it's as pretty and soft as its voice. But I'm getting sunburned, John. How hot a March day can get!"

"Only two more miles and good road all the way."

A few minutes more and Mary was set down at Centerville, "I'll be back about sunset," announced her husband as he drove off.

A very pleasant-faced woman answered the knock at the door. She had a shingle in her hand and several long strips of muslin over her arm. She smilingly explained that she didn't often meet people at the door with a shingle but that she was standing near the door when the knock came.

Mary, standing by the bed and removing hat and gloves, looked about her.

"What are you doing with that shingle and all this cotton and stuff, Mrs. Parkin?" she asked.

"Haven't you ever made a splint?"

"A splint? No indeed, I'm not equal to that."

"That's what I'm doing now. There's a boy with a broken arm in the office in the next room."

"Oh, your husband has his office here at the house."

"Yes, and it's a nuisance sometimes, too, but one gets used to it."

"I'll watch you and learn something new about the work of a doctor's wife."

"You'll learn then to have a lot of pillow slips and sheets on hand. Old or new, Dr. Parkin just tears them up when he gets in a hurry—it doesn't matter to him what goes."

The doctor's wife put cotton over the whole length of the shingle and wound the strips of muslin around it; then taking a needle and thread she stitched it securely. Mary sat in her chair watching the process with much interest. "You have made it thicker in some places than in others," she said.

"Yes; that is to fit the inequalities of the arm." Mary looked at her admiringly. "You are something of an artist," she observed.

Just as Mrs. Parkin finished it her husband appeared in the doorway.

"Is it done?" he asked.

"It's just finished."

"May I see you put it on, Doctor?" asked Mary, rising and coming forward.

"Why, good afternoon, Mrs. Blank. I'm glad to see you out here. Yes, come right in. How's the doctor?"

"Oh, he is well and happy—I think he expects to cut off a foot this afternoon."

A boy with a frightened look on his face stood in the doctor's office with one sleeve rolled up. The doctor adjusted the fracture, then applied the splint while his wife held it steady until he had made it secure. When the splint was in place and the boy had gone a messenger came to tell the doctor he was wanted six miles away.

About half an hour afterward a little black-eyed woman came in and said she wanted some more medicine like the last she took.

"The doctor's gone," said Mrs. Parkin, "and will not be back for several hours."

"Well, you can get it for me, can't you?"

"Do you know the name of it?"

"No, but I believe I could tell it if I saw it," said the patient, going to the doctor's shelves and looking closely at the bottles and phials with their contents of many colors. She took up a three-ounce bottle. "This is like the other bottle and I believe the medicine is just the same color. Yes, I'm sure it is," she said, holding it up to the light. Mary looked at her and then at Mrs. Parkin.

"I wouldn't like to risk it," said the latter lady.

"Oh, I'm not afraid. I don't want to wait until the doctor comes and I know this must be like the other. It's exactly the same color."

"My good woman," said Mary, "you *certainly* will not risk that. It might kill you."

"No, Mrs. Dawson, you must either wait till the doctor comes or come again," said Mrs. Parkin. The patient grumbled a little about having to make an extra trip and took her leave.

When the door had closed behind her Mary asked the other doctor's wife if she often had patients like that.

"Oh, yes. People come here when the doctor is away and either want me to prescribe for them or to prescribe for themselves."

"You don't do it, do you?"

"Sometimes I do, when I am perfectly sure what I am doing. Having the office here in the house so many years I couldn't help learning a few things."

"I wouldn't prescribe for anything or anybody. I'd be afraid of killing somebody." About an hour later Mary, looking out of the window, saw a wagon stopping at the gate. It contained a man and a woman and two well-grown girls.

"Hello!" called the man.

"People call you out instead of coming in. That is less trouble," observed Mary. The doctor's wife went to the door.

"Is Doc at home?"

"No, he has gone to the country."

"How soon will he be back?"

"Not before supper time, probably."

The man whistled, then looked at his wife and the two girls.

"Well, Sally," he said, "I guess we'd better git out and wait fur 'im."

"W'y, Pa, it'll be dark long before we git home, if we do."

"I can't help that. I'm not agoin' to drive eight miles tomorry or next day nuther."

"If ye'd 'a started two hour ago like I wanted ye to do, maybe Doc'd 'a been here and we c'd 'a been purty nigh home by this time."

"Shet up! I told ye I wasn't done tradin' then."

"It don't take *me* all day to trade a few aigs for a jug o' m'lasses an' a plug o' terbacker."

For answer the head of the house told his family to "jist roll out now." They rolled out and in a few minutes they had all rolled in. Mrs. Parkin made a heroic effort not to look inhospitable which made Mary's heroic effort not to look amused still more heroic.

When at last the afternoon was drawing to a close Mary went out into the yard to rest. She wished John would come. Hark! There is the ring of horses' hoofs down the quiet road. But these are white horses, John's are bays. She turns her head and looks into the west. Out in the meadow a giant oak-tree stands between her and the setting sun. Its upper branches are outlined against the grey cloud which belts the entire western horizon, while its lower branches are sharply etched against the yellow sky beneath the grey.

What a calm, beautiful sky it was!

She thought of some lines she had read more than once that morning ... a bit from George Eliot's Journal:

"How lovely to look into that brilliant distance and see the ship on the horizon seeming to sail away from the cold and dim world behind it right into the golden glory! I have always that sort of feeling when I look at sunset. It always seems to me that there in the west lies a land of light and warmth and love."

A carriage was now coming down the road at great speed. Mary saw it was her husband and went in to put on her things. In a few minutes more she was in the buggy and they were bound for home. It was almost ten o'clock when they got there. The trip had been so hard on the horses that all the spirit was taken out of them. The doctor, too, was exceedingly tired. "Forty-two miles is a long trip to make in an afternoon," he said.

"I hope Jack and Maggie are not up so late."

"It would be just like them to sit up till we came."

The buggy stopped; the door flew open and Jack and Maggie stood framed in the doorway with the leaping yellow firelight for a background.

# CHAPTER V.

Once in a while sympathy for a fellow mortal kept the doctor's wife an interested listener at the 'phone. Going, one morning, to speak to a friend about some little matter she heard her husband say:

"What is it, doctor?" A physician in a little town some ten or twelve miles distant, who had called Dr. Blank in consultation a few days before, was calling him.

"I think our patient is doing very well, but her heart keeps getting a little faster."

"How fast is it now?"

"About 120."

"But the disease is pretty well advanced now—that doesn't mean as much as it would earlier. But you might push a little on the brandy, or the strychnine—how much brandy have you given her since I saw her?"

"I have given her four ounces."

"Four ounces!"

"Yes."

"Four ounces in three days? I think you must mean four drachms."

"*Yes*. It *is* drachms. Four ounces *would* be fixing things up. I've been giving her digitalis; what do you think about that?"

"That's all right, but I think that strychnine would be a little better."

"Would you give her any aromatic spirits of ammonia?"

"Does she rattle?"

"A little."

"Then you might give her a little of that. And keep the room open and stick right to her and she ought to get along. Don't give her much to eat."

"Is milk all right?"

"Yes. You bet it is."

"All right then, doctor, I believe that's all. Good-bye."

On another occasion, Mary caught this fragment:

"She's so everlastin' sore that she just hollers and yells every time I go near her. Would you give her any more morphine?"

"Morphine's a thing you can't monkey with you know, Doctor. You want to be mighty careful about that."

"Yes. I know. How long will that morphine last?"

"That depends on how you use it. It won't last long if you use too much and neither will she."

"I mean how long will it last in the system?"

"O! Why, three or four hours."

"Well, I think she don't need no more medicine."

Mary smiled at the double negative and when she laughingly spoke of it that night her husband assured her that that doctor's singleness of purpose more than offset his doubleness of negative. That he was a fine fellow and a good physician just the same.

One morning in March just as the doctor arose from the breakfast table he was called to the 'phone.

"Is this Dr. Blank?"

"Yes."

"Doctor, will it hurt the baby to bathe it every morning? I've been doing that but some of the folks around here say I oughtn't to do it; they say it isn't good for a baby to bathe it so often."

The doctor answered solemnly, "The baby's fat and healthy isn't it?"

"Yes, sir."

"And pretty?"

"Yes, *sir.*"

"Likes to see its mamma?"

"You *know* it."

"Likes to see its papa?"

"He does that!" said the young mother.

"Then ask me next fall if it will hurt to bathe the baby every morning."

"All right, Doctor," laughed the baby's mamma.

"The fools are not all dead yet," said John, as he took his hat and departed. On the step he turned back and put his head in at the door. "Keep an ear out, Mary. I'm likely to be away from the office a good bit this morning."

An hour later a call came. Mary put the ear that was "out" to the receiver:

"It's on North Adams street."

"All right. I'll be out there after awhile," said her husband's placid voice.

"Don't wait too long. He may die before you git here."

"No, he won't. I'll be along pretty soon."

"Well, come just as quick as you can."

"All right," and the listener knew that it might be along toward noon before he got there.

About eleven o'clock the 'phone rang sharply.

"Is this Dr. Blank's house?"

"Yes."

"Is he there?"

"I saw him pass here about twenty minutes ago. I'm sure he'll be back to the office in a little bit."

"My land! I've been here three or four times. Looks like I'd ketch him *some* time."

"You are at the office then? If you will sit down and wait just a little while, he will be in."

"I come six miles to see him. I supposed of course he'd be in *some* time," grumbled the voice (of course a woman's).

"But when he is called to visit a patient he must go, you know," explained Mary.

"Y-e-s," admitted the voice reluctantly. "Well, I'll wait here a little while longer."

Ten minutes later Mary rang the office. Her husband replied.

"How long have you been back, John?"

"O, five or ten minutes."

"Did you find a woman waiting for you?"

"No."

- 38 -

"Well, I assured her you'd be there in a few minutes and she said she'd wait."

"Do you know who she was?"

"No. Some one from the country. She said she came six miles to see you and she supposed you'd be in your office *some* time, and that sometime was mightily emphatic."

"O, yes, I know now. She'll be in again," laughed the doctor and Mary felt relieved, for in the querulous tones of the disappointed woman she had read disapproval of the doctor and of herself too, as the partner not only of his joys and sorrows, but of his laggard gait as well. The people who wait for a doctor are not apt to consider that a good many more may be waiting for him also at that particular moment of time.

# CHAPTER VI.

One of the most discouraging things I have encountered is a great blank silence. The doctor asks his wife to keep a close watch on the telephone for a little while, and leaves the office. Pretty soon it rings and she goes to answer it.

"Hello?" Silence. "What is it?" More silence. She knows that "unseen hands or spirits" did not ring that bell. She knows perfectly well that there is a listening ear at the other end of the line. But you cannot converse with silence any more than you can speak to a man you meet on the street if he purposely looks the other way.

Mary knew that the listening ear belonged to someone who recognized that it was the wife who answered instead of the doctor, and therefore kept silent. She smiled and hung up the receiver—sorry not to be able to help her husband and to give the needed information to the patient.

But when this had happened several times she thought of a more satisfactory way of dealing with the situation. She would take down the receiver and ask, "What is it?" She would wait a perceptible instant and then say distinctly and pleasantly, "Doctor Blank will be out of the office for about twenty minutes. He asked me to tell you." That never failed to bring an answer, a hasty, shame-voiced, "Oh, I—well—thank you, Mrs. Blank, I'll call again, then."

The doctor's absence from town has its telephonic puzzles. One day during Dr. Blank's absence his wife was called to the 'phone.

"Mrs. Blank, a telegram has just come for the doctor. What must I do with it?" It was the man at the office who put the question.

"Do you know what it is, or where it's from?"

"I asked the operator and he says it's from Mr. Slocum, who is in Cincinnati. He telegraphed the doctor to go and see his wife who is sick."

"Well, take it over to Dr. Brown's office and ask him to go and see her."

About half an hour later the thought of the telegram came into her mind. "I wonder if he found Dr. Brown in. I'd better find out."

She rang the office. "Did you find Dr. Brown in?"

"Yes, he was there."

"And you gave the message to him?"

"Yes, he took it."

"I hope he went right down?"

"No, he said he wouldn't go."

"Wouldn't go!" exclaimed Mary, much astonished.

"He said he knew Slocum and he was in all probability drunk when he sent the message."

"Why, what a queer conclusion to arrive at. The doctor may be right but I think we ought to know."

"I called up their house after I came back from Dr. Brown's office, but nobody answered. So she can't be very sick or she'd be at home."

Mary put up the receiver hesitatingly. She was not satisfied about this matter. She went about her work, but her thoughts were on the message and the sick wife. Suddenly she thought of something—the Slocum children were in school. The mother had not been able to get to the 'phone to answer it. The thought of her lying there alone and helpless was too much. Mary went swiftly to the telephone and called the office.

"Johnson, you have to pass Mrs. Slocum's on your way to dinner. I think she may have been too ill to go to the 'phone. Please stop and find out something definite."

"All right."

"And let me know as soon as you can. If she isn't sick don't tell her anything about the telegram. Think up some excuse as you go along for coming in, in case all is well."

In about twenty minutes the expected summons came.

"Well, I stopped, Mrs. Blank."

"What did you find?"

"Well, I found a hatchet close to Slocum's gate."

"How lucky!"

"I took it in to ask if it was theirs."

"Was it?"

"No, it wasn't."

"Who told you so?"

"Mrs. Slocum, herself, and she's about the healthiest looking invalid I've seen lately."

"I'm much relieved. Thank you, Johnson." And as she left the 'phone she meditated within herself, "Verily, the tender thoughtfulness of the husband drunk exceedeth that of the husband sober."

When night came and Mary was preparing for bed she thought, "It will be very unpleasant to be called up only to tell people the doctor is not here." She rose, went to the 'phone and called central.

"This is Mrs. Blank, central. If anyone should want the doctor tonight, or for the next two nights, please say he is out of town and will not be home until Saturday."

Then with a delicious sense of freedom she went to bed and slept as sweetly as in the long-ago when the telephone was a thing undreamed of.

The ting-a-ling-ling-ling—came as Mary was pouring boiling water into the teapot, just before six on a cool July evening. The maid was temporarily absent and Mary had been getting supper in a very leisurely way when she saw her husband step up on the porch. Then her leisure was exchanged for hurry. The doctor's appearance before meal time was the signal to which she responded automatically—he had to catch a train—someone must have him right away, or what not? She must not keep him waiting a minute. She pushed the teapot back on the stove and went swiftly to the 'phone.

"Is this Dr. Blank's office?" asked a disturbed feminine voice.

"No, his residence. He is here. Wait a minute, please, and I will call him."

She hurried out to the porch, "Isn't papa here?" she asked of her small boy sitting there.

"He *was*."

"Well, where is he now?"

"I don't know where he is."

Provoking! She hurried back. He must be in the garden. An occasional impulse to hoe sometimes came over him (especially if the day happened to be Sunday).

In the kitchen her daughter stood at a table cutting the bread for supper. "Go quick, and see if papa's in the garden. Tell him to come to the 'phone at once."

Then she hurried back to re-assure the waiting one. But what could she tell her? Perhaps the doctor was not in the garden. She rushed out and beat her daughter in the race toward it. She sent her voice ahead, "John!" she called.

"Yes."

"Come to the 'phone this minute." Back she ran. Would she still be waiting?

"Hello."

"Hello."

"Yes, the doctor's here. He's in the garden but will be in in just a minute. Hold the 'phone please."

"Very well, thank you."

It was a minute and a half before the doctor got there.

"Hello." No answer.

"Hello!" Silence.

"*Hello!*" Still no reply. The doctor rang sharply for central.

"Who was calling me a minute ago."

"I don't know—we can't keep track of everybody who calls."

The doctor hung up the receiver with an explosive monosyllable. Mary's patience was giving out too. "She couldn't wait one half minute. I told her you would be here in a minute and it took you a minute and a half."

"She may be waiting at the office, I'll go down there."

"I wouldn't do it," said Mary, warmly. "It's much easier for her to stay a half minute at the 'phone than for you to tramp back to the office."

But he went. As his wife went back to the kitchen her daughter called, "Mother, did you take the loaf of bread in there with you?"

"Why, no."

"Well, it's not on the table where I was cutting it when you sent me after father."

"It's on the floor!" shouted the small boy, peering through the window. "*I* won't eat any of it!"

"Don't, exquisite child," said his sister, stooping over to recover the loaf, dropped in her haste. Ting-a-ling-ling-ling. Mary went.

"Isn't the doctor coming?"

"He came. He called repeatedly, but got no reply."

"I was right here with my ear to the 'phone the whole time."

"He concluded it might be someone waiting for him at the office, so he has gone down there."

"I'm not there. I'm here at home."

"Hello," broke in the doctor's voice.

"O, here you are!"

"Doctor, I've been taking calomel today and then I took some salts and I thoughtlessly dissolved them in some lemonade I had handy!"

A solemn voice asked, "Have you made your will?"

A little giggle before the patient said "No."

"You'll have plenty of time. You needn't hurry about it."

"You don't think it will hurt me then?"

"No. Not a bit."

"I was afraid the acid might salivate me."

"Yes, that's an old and popular idea. But it won't."

"That sounds good, Doctor. I was awfully scared. Much obliged. Good-bye."

A week or two after the above incident the doctor was seated at his dinner, a leisurely Sunday dinner. The telephone called and he rose and went to it. The usual hush fell upon the table in order that he might hear.

"Is this Dr. Blank?"

"Yes."

"Well, Doctor, this is Mrs. Abner. Would it be too much trouble for you to step into Hall's and ask them to send me up a quart of ice-cream for dinner?"

"Certainly not. A quart?"

"Yes, please. I'm sorry to bother you with it. They ought to have a 'phone."

"No trouble."

The doctor hung up the receiver and reached for his hat.

"Why, John, you surely can finish your dinner before you go!" exclaimed Mary.

"Then I'd spoil Mrs. Abner's dinner."

"Mrs. Abner!"

"Yes, she wants a quart of ice-cream for dinner."

"I'd like to know what *you've* got to do with it," said Mary tartly.

"She thinks I'm at the office."

"And the office is next door to Hall's and Hall's have no 'phone," said Mary smiling. "Of course you must go. Wouldn't Mrs. Abner feel mortified though if she knew you had to leave your home in the midst of dinner to order her ice-cream. But do hurry back, John."

"Maybe I'd better stay there till the dinner hour is well over," laughed John. "Every now and then someone wants me to step into Hall's and order up something."

He went good-naturedly away and his wife looked after him marveling, but withal admiring.

The doctor and his wife had been slumbering peacefully for an hour or two. Then came a loud ring and they were wide awake at once.

"That wasn't the telephone, John, it was the door-bell."

The doctor got into his dressing-gown and went to the door.

His wife heard a man's voice, then her husband reply, then the door shut. She lay back on her pillow but it was evident John was not coming back. She must have dozed, for it seemed to her a long time had gone by when she started to hear a noise in the other room. John had not yet got off.

"You have to go some place, do you?" she called.

"Yes,—just a little way. Look out for the 'phone, Mary. I think I'll have to go down to Hanson's tonight, to meet the stork."

"But how can I get word to you? They have no 'phone or that man wouldn't have come after you."

"Well, I have promised Hanson and I'll have to go there. If he 'phones before I get back tell him he'll have to come down to Stetson's after me. Or, you might wake one of the boys and send him over."

"I'd rather try to wake Rip Van Winkle," said Mary, in a tone that settled it.

In about an hour the doctor was back and snuggling down under the covers.

"They've got a fine boy over to Stetson's," he announced to his sleepy wife.

"They have!" she exclaimed, almost getting awake. Again they slept.

Ting-a-ling-ling-ling. Ting-a-ling-ling-ling. Ting-a-ling-ling-ling.

"That's Hanson," exclaimed the doctor springing up and groping his way to the 'phone.

"Yes."

"Out where?"

"Smith's on Parks avenue?.... *Not* Smith's?.... I understand—a little house farther down that street..... Yes, I'll come..... O, as soon as I can dress and get there."

Mary heard, but when he had gone, was soon in a deep sleep.

By and by she found herself flinging off the covers and hurrying guiltily toward the summoning tyrant, her subconscious self telling her that this was the third peal.

"Hello."

"Is the doctor there, Mrs. Blank?"

"No, he is over at Stetson's. He said if you 'phoned to tell you you would have to come there as they have no 'phone."

"Wait a minute, Mrs. Blank," said the voice of central, "some one is trying to speak—"

"What have I said!" thought Mary suddenly, thoroughly awake. "He got back from Stetson's and went to another place. But I don't know what place nor where it is."

The kindly voice of central went on:

"It's the doctor who is talking, Mrs. Blank. I understand now. He says if that message comes you are to 'phone him at James Smith's on Parks avenue."

Mary looked at the clock. "So he's been there all this time. That stork is a little too busy tonight," she thought as she went shivering back to bed.

Toward daylight she was roused by the return of her husband, who announced a new daughter in the world and then they went to sleep. The next morning she said, "John, I've just thought of something. Why didn't you have central 'phone you at Smith's if Hanson called and save me all that bother?"

"I guess it's because I'm so used to bothering you Mary, that I didn't think of it."

Mary was upstairs cleaning house most vigorously when the ring came. She stopped and listened. It came again—three. She set the dust pan down and went.

"I'll have to be out for an hour or more, Mary," said the doctor.

"I heard that sigh," he laughed, "but it won't be very hard to sort of keep an ear on the 'phone, will it? Johnson may get in soon and then it won't be necessary."

"Very well, then, John," and she went upstairs, leaving the doors open behind her.

She had just reached the top when she had to turn about and retrace her steps.

"Hello." No answer.

"Is someone calling Dr. Blank's house or office?"

"I rang your 'phone by mistake," said central. Mary trudged up the stairs again. "This is more tiresome than cleaning house," she said to herself as she went along.

In twenty minutes the summons came. She leaned her broom against the wall and went down.

"O, this is Mrs. Blank. I'm very sorry to have put you to this trouble—I wanted the doctor."

She recognized the voice of her old pastor for whom she had a most kindly regard.

"He is out, but will be back within half an hour now, Mr. Rutledge."

"Thank you, I'll call again, but I wonder that you knew my voice." Mary laughed.

"I haven't heard it for awhile, but maybe I'll be at church next Sunday, if minding the telephone doesn't make me feel too wicked."

"It's the wicked that church is for—come by all means."

"I didn't mean to detain you, Mr. Rutledge. It is restful, though, after dragging one's weary feet down to the 'phone to hear something beside all the ills that flesh is heir to. Come to see us soon—one day next week."

Once more she wended her way upstairs and in about fifteen minutes came the ting-a-ling-a-ling-a-ling. "I surrender!" she declared.

When she had gone down and put the receiver to her ear her husband's voice spoke kindly,

"I'm back, Mary, you're released."

"Thank you, John, you are very thoughtful," and she smiled as she took off her sun-bonnet and sat herself down. "Not another time will I climb those stairs this morning."

Mary sat one evening dreamily thinking about them—these messages that came every day, every day!

Doctor, will it hurt Jennie to eat some tomatoes this morning—she craves them so?

Will is a great deal better. Can he have some ice-cream for dinner?

I can hardly manage Henry any longer, Doctor, he's determined he *will* have more to eat. Can I begin giving him a little more today?

Lemonade won't hurt Helen, will it? She wants some.

Doctor, I forget how many drops of that clear medicine I am to give..... Ten, you say? Thank you.

Dr. Blank, is it after meals or before that the dark medicine is to be given..... I thought so, but I wanted to be sure.

We are out of those powders you left. Do you think we will need any more?.... Then I'll send down for them.

How long will you be in the office this morning, Doctor?...... Very well, I'll be down in about an hour. I want you to see my throat.

You wanted me to let you know how Johnny is this morning. I don't think he has any fever now and he slept all night, so I guess you won't need to come down today.

Dr. Blank, I've got something coming on my finger. Do you suppose it's a felon?.... You can tell better when you see it?.... Well, I suppose you can. I'll be down at the office pretty soon and then I want you to tell me it's *not* a felon.

Mary seems a good deal better this morning, but she still has that pain in her side.

Doctor, I don't believe Joe is as well as he was last night. I think you had better come down.

As these old, old stories came leisurely into Mary's thoughts the telephone rang three times. She rose from her chair before the fire and went to answer it.

"Is this Dr. Blank's office?"

"No, his residence."

"Is the doctor there?"

"No, but he will be down on the seven o'clock train."

"And it's now not quite six. This is Mr. Andrews."

Mary knew the name and the man.

"My wife is sick and I want to get a pint of alcohol for her."

"An old subterfuge," thought Mary, "I'm afraid he wants it for himself."
She knew that he was often under its influence.

"I can't get it without a prescription from a physician, you know. She needs
it right away."

"The thirst is on him," thought our listener, pityingly.

The voice went on, "Mrs. Blank, couldn't you just speak to the druggist
about it so I could get it right away?"

"Mr. Andrews," she said hastily, "the druggist would pay no attention to
me. I'm not a physician, you know. The doctor will be here in an hour—see
him," and she hurried the receiver into its place, anxious to get away from
it. This was a story that was entirely new to her. Never before had she been
asked to procure a prescription for alcohol or any of its attendant spirits.
She liked the old stories best.

The doctor had been to the city and had got home at four o'clock in the
morning. He had had to change cars in the night and consequently had had
little sleep. When the door-bell rang his wife awakened instantly at the
expected summons and rose to admit him. In a little while both were fast
asleep. The wife, about a half hour later, found herself struggling to speak
to somebody about something, she did not know what. But when the
second long peal came from the 'phone she was fully awakened. How she
hated to rouse the slumberer at her side.

"John," she called softly. He did not move.

"John!" a little louder. He stirred slightly, but slept on.

"John, *John!*"

"Huh-h?"

"The telephone."

He threw back the covers, and rising, stumbled to the 'phone.

"Hello."

The voice of a little boy came to his half-awakened ear.

"*Say*, Pa, *I* can't sell these papers an' git through in time fer school."

"Yes, you *can*!" roared a voice. "You jist want to fool around." The doctor went back to bed.

"Wasn't the message for you?" inquired his wife. "What a shame to rouse you from your sleep for nothing."

The doctor told her what the message was and was back in slumberland in an incredibly short space of time. Not so his wife. She was too thoroughly awake at last and dawn was beginning to peep around the edges of the window shades. She would not court slumber now but would lie awake with her own thoughts which were very pleasant thoughts this morning. By and by she rose softly, dressed and went out onto the veranda and looked long into the reddening eastern sky. Ever since she could remember she had felt this keen delight at the aspect of the sky in the very early morning. She stood for awhile, drinking in the beauty and the peacefulness of it all. Then she went in to her awakening household, glad that the little boy had 'phoned his "Pa" and by some means had got her too.

One midsummer night a tiny ringing came faintly and pleasantly into Mary's dreams. Not till it came the second or third time did she awaken to what it was. Then she sat up in bed calling her husband, who had just awakened too and sprung out of bed. Dazed, he stumbled about and could not find his way. With Mary's help he got his bearings and the next minute his thunderous "Hello" greeted her ears.

"Yes."

"Worse tonight? In what way?"

An instant's silence. "Mrs. Brownson?" Silence. "Mrs. Brownson!" Silence.

"Damn that woman! She's rung off."

"Well, don't swear into the 'phone, John. It's against the rules. Besides, she might hear you."

The doctor was growling his way to his clothes.

"I suppose I've got to go down there," was all the answer he made. When he was dressed and the screen had banged behind him after the manner of screens, Mary settled herself to sleep which came very soon. But she was soon routed out of it. She went to the 'phone, expecting to hear a querulous woman's voice asking, "Has the doctor started yet?" and her lips were framing the old and satisfactory reply, "Yes, he must be nearly there now," when a man's voice asked, "Is this Dr. Blank's residence?"

"Yes."

"Is the doctor there?"

"No, but he will be back in about twenty minutes."

"Will you please tell him to come to J. H. Twitchell's?"

"Yes, I'll send him right down."

"Thank you."

She went back to her bed room then, turning, retraced her steps. The doctor could come home by way of Twitchell's as their home was not a great distance from the Brownson's.

She rang the Brownson's and after a little while a voice answered.

"Is this Mrs. Brownson?"

"Yes."

"May I speak to Dr. Blank. I think he must be there now."

"He's been here. He's gone home."

Mary knew by the voice that its owner had not enjoyed getting out of bed. "I wonder how she would like to be in my place," she thought, smiling. She dared not trust herself to her pillow. She might fall asleep and not waken when her husband came in. She wondered what time it was. Up there on the wall the clock was ticking serenely away—she had only to turn the button beside her to find out. But she did not turn it. In the sweet security of the dark she felt safe. In one brief flash of light some prowling burglar might discover her.

She sat down by the open window and looked up into the starlit sky. They were out tonight in countless numbers. Over there toward the northwest, lying along the tops of the trees was the Great Dipper. Wasn't it? Surely that particular curve in the handle was not to be found in any other constellation. She tried to see the Dipper itself but a cherry tree near her window blotted it out. Bend and peer as she might the branches intervened. It was tantalizing. She rose irresolute. Should she step out doors where the cherry tree would not be in the way? Not for a thousand dippers! She walked to another window. That view shut even the handle out. She looked for the Pleiades. They were not in the section of sky visible from the window where she stood. She turned and listened. Did she hear footsteps down the walk? She ought to be hearing her husband's by this time. He could not be walking at his usual gait. There he came! She went to the door looked through the screen and halted him as he drew near the steps.

"John, you'll have to take another trip. Mr. Twitchell has 'phoned for you."

He turned and was soon out of sight. "Now! I can go to bed with a clear conscience," and Mary sought her pillow. But she had better stay awake until he had time to get there lest Mr. Twitchell should 'phone again. In five or ten minutes the danger would be over. She waited. At last she closed her eyes to sleep. But what would be the use? In twenty minutes more her husband would come in and rouse her out of it. She had better just keep awake till he got back. And the next thing Mary heard was a snore. She opened her eyes to find it was broad daylight and her husband was sleeping soundly beside her.

# CHAPTER VII.

One afternoon in June Mary went into her husband's office.

"Has *The Record* come?" she asked.

"Yes, it's on the table in the next room."

She went into the adjoining room and seated herself by the table. Taking up *The Record*, she turned to the editorial page, but before she could begin reading she heard a voice in the office say, "How do you do, Doctor?"

"How do you do, Mr. Jenkins. Take a seat."

"No, I guess I'll not sit down. I just wanted to get—a prescription."

"The baby's better, isn't it?"

"Oh, the baby's all right, but I want a prescription for myself."

"What sort of prescription?"

"I have to take a long ride in the morning, driving cattle, and I want a prescription for a pint of whiskey."

Mary listened for her husband's reply. It came.

"Jenkins, I have taken many a long ride through dust and heat, through rain and snow and storm, and I never yet have had to take any whiskey along."

"Well, I have a little trouble with my heart and—"

"The trouble's in your head. If you'd throw away that infernal pipe—"

"Oh, it's no use to lecture me on that any more."

"Very well, your tobacco may be worth more to you than your heart."

"Well, will you give me that prescription?"

"Certainly I won't. You don't need whiskey and you'll not get it from me."

"Go to h-ll!"

"All right, I'll meet *you* there." At which warm farewell between these two good friends, Mary leaned back in her chair and laughed silently. Then she mused: "People will not be saved from themselves. If only they would be, how much less of sin and sickness and sorrow there would be in the world."

Presently the doctor came in.

"I have a trip to make tonight, Mary. How would you like a star-light drive?" Mary said she would like it very much indeed.

Accordingly, at sunset the doctor drove up and soon they were out in the open country. Chatting of many things they drove along and by and by Mary's eyes were attracted to a beautiful castle up in the clouds in the west, on a great golden rock jutting out into the blue. Far below was a grand woman's form in yellow floating robes. She stood with face upturned and arms extended in an attitude of sorrow as if she had been banished from her father's house.

There comes the father now. Slowly, majestically, an old man with flowing beard of gold moves toward the edge of the great rock. Now he has reached it. He bends his head and looks below. The attitude of the majestic woman has changed to that of supplication. And now the father stretches down forgiving arms and the queenly daughter bows her head against the mighty wall and weeps in gladness. Now castle and rock, father and daughter slowly interchange places and vanish from her sight. The gold turns to crimson, then fades to gray. Just before her up there in the clouds is a huge lion, couchant. See! he is going to spring across the pale blue chasm to the opposite bank. If he fails he will come right down into the road—"Oh!"

"What is it?" asked the doctor, looking around, and Mary told him with a rather foolish smile.

The twilight deepened into dusk and the notes of a whippoorwill came to them from a distance. "You and I must have nothing but sweet thoughts right now, John, because then we'll get to keep them for a year." She quoted:

"'Tis said that whatever sweet feeling

May be throbbing within the fond heart,

When listening to a whippoorwill s-pieling,

For a twelvemonth will never depart."

"Spieling doesn't seem specially in the whippoorwill's line."

"It's *exactly* in his line. Years ago when I was a little girl he proved it. One evening at dusk I was sitting in an arbor when he, not suspecting my presence, alighted within a few feet of me and began his song. It was wonderfully interesting to watch his little throat puff and puff with the notes as they poured forth, but the thing that astounded me was the length of time he sang without ever pausing for breath. And so he is a genuine spieler. I will add, however, that the line is 'When listening to a whippoorwill *singing.*' But my literary conscience will never let me rhyme *singing* with *feeling*, hence the sudden change."

"Now I'll speak *my* piece," announced the doctor:

> "De frogs in de pon' am a singin' all de night;
>
> Wid de hallelujah campmeetin' tune;
>
> An' dey all seem to try wid deir heart, soul and might
>
> To tell us ob de comin' of de June."

"*Aren't* they having a hallelujah chorus over in that meadow, though!"

Darkness settled over the earth. The willow trees, skirting the road for a little distance, lifted themselves in ghostly tracery against the starlit sky. A soft breeze stirred their branches like the breath of a gentle spirit abiding there. They passed a cozy farmhouse nestled down among tall trees. Through the open door they could see a little white-robed figure being carried to bed in its father's arms, while the mother crooned a lullaby over the cradle near.

For a long time they drove in silence. Mary knew that her husband was in deep thought. Of what was he thinking? The pretty home scene in the farm house had sent him into a reverie. He went back five or six years to a bright spring day. He was sitting alone in his office when an old man, a much respected farmer, came in slowly, closed the door behind him and sat down. The doctor who knew him quite well saw that he was troubled and asked if there was anything he could do for him. The old man leaned his head on his hand but did not reply. It seemed that no words would come in which to tell his errand.

Puzzled and sympathetic the doctor sat silent and waited. In a little while the farmer drew his chair very near to that of the doctor's and said in a low voice, "Doctor, I'm in deep trouble. I come to you because you are one of my best friends. You have a chance to prove it now such as you never had before in all the years you've been our doctor."

"Tell me your trouble and if I can help you, I will certainly do so."

"It's Mary. She's gone wrong, and the disgrace will kill her mother if she finds it out."

For an instant the doctor did not speak; then he asked, "Are you sure that this is true?"

"Yes. She came to me last night and nestled down in my arms, just as she's done every night since she was a baby. She cried like her heart would break and then she said, 'Father, I *must* tell you, but don't tell mother'; and then she told me."

The old man, white and trembling, looked beseechingly at the doctor.

"Doctor, this must not be. You must stop it before there is any breath of scandal. Oh, for a minute last night I wanted to kill her."

The doctor's face was stern. "If you had killed her your crime would have been far less hellish than the one you ask me to commit."

The old man bowed his head upon his hands. "You will not help me," he groaned.

The doctor rose and walked the floor. "No, sir," he said, "I will not stain my soul with murder for you or any other man." He went to the window and stood looking out upon the street below. Presently he said, "Mr. Stirling, will you come here a minute?" The old man rose and went. "Do you see that little boy skipping along down there?"

"Yes, I see him."

"If I should go down these stairs, seize him and dash his brains out against that building, what would you think of me?"

"I'd think you were a devil."

"Yet he would have a chance for his life. He could cry out, or the passersby might see me and interpose, while that you ask me to destroy is—"

"There's one thing I'll do," said the old man fiercely. "I'll kill Ben Morely before this day is over!" He seized his hat and started toward the door.

"Wait a minute!" said the doctor quickly. "It's Ben Morely is it? I know him. I would not have thought him capable of this."

"He's been coming to see Mary steady for more than a year and they were to have been married three months ago but they quarreled and Mary told me last night that he was going away the last of this week. She is as good and sweet a girl as ever lived. She never kept company with anybody else and she thought the world of him. The damned villain has got around her with his honey words and now he proposes to leave her to face it alone. But I'll kill him as sure as the sun shines."

"Sit down," said the doctor, laying a hand on the excited man's arm and forcing him into a chair.

"Let me tell you what to do. Young Morely's father is a good and sensible man and will take the right view of it. Go straight to him and tell him all about it and my word for it, he will see that they are married right away. He is able to help them along and will make it to his son's advantage to stay here rather than go away. He will advise him right. Have no fear." The old man wrung the doctor's hand in silence and went out.

Several days later the doctor was looking over the papers published in the town and read in the list of marriage licenses the names, "Benjamin Morely, aged twenty-four, Mary Stirling, aged eighteen."

And that is why the scene in the farmhouse this summer night had sent him back into the past, for it was the home of Benjamin and Mary Morely, and it was a happy home. These two lives had come together and flowed on in such harmony and helpfulness and rectitude before the world that the stain had been wiped out. For a merciless world can be merciful sometimes if it will only stop to remember that long ago a compassionate Voice said, Go and sin no more.

The doctor's reverie came to an end for he had reached his destination—a large white house standing very close to the road.

"Don't talk to me while you are hitching the horse," Mary whispered, "then they won't know there is anyone with you. I don't want to go in—I want to see the moon come up."

The doctor took his case and went inside. Mary sat in the buggy and listened. The neighing of a horse far down the road and the barking of a dog in the distance were the only sounds she heard. How still and cool it was after the heat of the day. A wandering breeze brought the sweet perfume of dewy clover fields. She looked across the intervening knoll to the east. The tree that crowned its summit stood outlined against the brightening sky. She was sitting very near the open kitchen window and now saw the family taking their places around the supper table. She felt a little uncomfortable and as if she were trespassing on their privacy. But they did not know of her proximity and she could only sit still in the friendly cover of the darkness. How good the ham smelled and the potatoes and the coffee.

A pretty home-scene!

The father at the head of the table, the mother opposite with four sturdy boys between them, two on each side. The father looked around the board. Stillness settled down upon them, and then he bowed his head. The mother, too, bowed her head. The boys looked down.

"Our heavenly Father, we thank Thee for these evening blessings—" the boys looked up and four forks started simultaneously for the meat platter. Every fork impaled its slice. Mary gasped. She crammed her handkerchief into her mouth to shut off the laughter that almost shouted itself before she could stop it.

The oldest boy, a burly fellow of fifteen, looked astonished and then sheepish. The other three looked defiance at him. Each sat erect in perfect silence and held his slice to the platter with a firm hand. Mary, almost suffocating with laughter which *must* be suppressed, watched anxiously for the denouement. The blessing went on. The boys evidently knew all its stages. As it advanced there was a tightening of the tension and at the welcome "amen" there was a grand rake-off.

At the commotion of the sudden swipe the father and mother looked up in amazement.

"Boys, boys! what do you mean!" exclaimed the mother.

"We got even with Mr. Jake that time." It was the second boy who spoke.

"We got *ahead* of him," said the third. "He didn't get the biggest piece this time."

"No, *I* got it myself," said the fourth.

"Well, I'm scandalized," said the mother, looking across the table at her husband.

"Well, Mother, I'll tell you how it was," said the second boy. "Last night I looked up before Father was through with the blessing and I saw Jake with his fork in the biggest piece of ham. You and Father didn't notice and so he was *it*. I'll bet he's been at it a good while, too."

"I've not, either," said the accused.

"I told Bob and Jim about it and we concluded *we'd* take a hand in it tonight."

"Well, let this be the last of it," said the father with mild sternness. "We'll try to have ham enough for all of you without sneaking it. If not, Jacob can have his mother's share and mine."

The trio of boys grinned triumphantly at the discomfited Jake, then, the little flurry over, all fell to eating with a will.

The doctor's voice came to Mary from the room of the patient.

"You're worth a dozen dead women yet," it said. Then a high pitched woman's voice, "I'll tell you what Mary Ann says she thinks about it."

"Has she been here today?" If Mary Ann had been there the unfavorable condition of the patient was explained.

"Yes, she just went away. She says she believes you're just keepin' Ellen down so you can get a big bill out of her."

The doctor was fixing up powders and went placidly on till he got through, then he said "Mary Ann has a better opinion of me than I thought she had. It takes a mighty good doctor to do that. That's a very old song but there are a few people in the world that like to sing it yet. They don't know that there isn't a doctor in the world that knows enough to do a thing like that even if he wanted to. Nature would beat him every time if they gave her a chance."

Mary heard the doctor give his instructions and then he came out. As they drove off she asked, "You came pretty near catching a tartar, didn't you?"

"Oh, that one is all right. It's her sister that's always raising the devil."

"Look! isn't she lovely, John?"

"Isn't who lovely?" asked the doctor, looking back at the house in some surprise.

"The gentle Shepherdess of Night," Mary answered, her eyes on the moon just rising over the distant treetops.

"She's getting ready to 'lead her flocks through the fields of blue.'"

"How very poetical we are."

"Only an echo from a little song I used to sing when I was a little girl."

"Get up, my steeds," urged the doctor, "we must be getting back"; and they sped swiftly homeward through the soft summer night.

# CHAPTER VIII.

Ting-a-ling-ling-ling. Ting-a-ling-ling-ling. Ting-a-ling-ling-ling.

"Hello."

"Is this the doctor's office?"

"This is his residence."

"Pshaw! I wanted his *office*."

"The doctor 'phoned me about ten minutes ago that he would be out for half an hour and asked me to answer the 'phone in his absence," Mary explained, pleasantly.

"Oh," said the voice, somewhat mollified, "I'll just call him up when he gets back. You say he'll be back in half an hour?"

"In about that time."

She went back to her work, which happened to be upstairs this morning, leaving the doors ajar behind her that she might hear the 'phone. In two minutes she was summoned down.

"What is it?"

"Is this the doctor's office?"

"No, the residence."

"I rang for the office, sorry to have troubled you, Mrs. Blank," said a man's voice.

"We are connected and when the doctor is out he expects me to be bell-boy," said Mary, recognizing the voice.

"I see. Will you please tell the doctor when he comes that my little boy is sick this morning and I want him to come down. Will he be back soon?"

"In a few minutes, I think."

She sat down by the fire. No use to go back upstairs till she had delivered the message. This was a pleasing contrast to the other; Mr. Owen had volunteered his message as if she really had a right to know and deliver it.

Ting-a-ling-ling-ling. Ting-a-ling-ling-ling. Mary felt reluctant to answer it— it sounded so like the first. And it was not the house call this time, but two rings which undeniably meant the office. But she must be true to the trust reposed in her. She went to the 'phone and softly taking down the receiver, listened; perhaps the doctor had got back and would answer it himself. Fervently she hoped so. But there was only silence at her ear, and the ever present far-off clack of attenuated voices. The silence seemed to bristle. But there was nothing for our listener to do but thrust herself into it.

"Hello," she said, very gently.

"O, I've got *you* again, have I! I *know* I rung the office this time, for I looked in the book to see. How does it happen I get the house?" Ill temper was manifest in every word.

"The office and residence are connected," explained Mary, patiently, "and when the 'phone rings while the doctor is out, he asks me to answer it for him."

"I don't see what good *that* does."

"It doesn't do any good when people do not care to leave a message," said Mary quietly.

"Well, I'd ruther deliver my message to *him*."

"Certainly. And I would much rather you would. I can at least say about what time he expects to return."

"You said awhile ago he'd be back in half an hour and he's not back *yet*."

The doctor's wife knew that she was held responsible for the delay. She smiled and glanced at the clock.

"It is just three minutes past the half hour," she said.

"Well, we're in an awful hurry for him. I'll ring agin d'reckly."

In five minutes a ring came again. Surely he would be there now, thought his wife, but she must go to the 'phone. She listened. Silence. Then the bell pealed sharply forth again. She decided to change her tactics and put the other woman on the defensive:

"Well!" she said impatiently, "I'm *very* sorry to have to answer you again but—"

"Is the doctor there?" asked a sweet, new voice. "Pardon me for interrupting you, but I'm very anxious."

"He will be at the office in just a few minutes," Mary answered, very gently indeed. She realized now that one cannot "monkey" with the telephone.

"Will you please tell him to come at once?" and she gave the street and number.

"I shall send him at once."

"Thank you, good-bye."

Before Mary could seat herself, the expected ring came in earnest. She answered it meekly.

"O, good gracious! hain't he got there yet—?"

"Not yet," said Mary, offering nothing further.

"Well, I've jist *got* to have a doctor. I'll git some one else." The threat in the tone made our listener smile.

"I think it would be a good thing to do," she said.

A pause. Then a voice with softening accents.

"But I'd lots ruther have Dr. Blank." No reply.

"Are ye there yit, Mrs. Blank?"

"Yes. I am here."

"He'll surely be back in a little bit now, won't he?"

"I think so."

"Won't *you* tell 'im to come down to Sairey Tucker's? I'm her sister and she's bad sick."

"If you will tell me where you live I will send him."

"He knows—he's been here."

"Very well," and she rang off.

With three messages hanging over her head and her conscience, she could not go upstairs to her work. She must dawdle about at this or that 'till the doctor returned. After awhile she went to the 'phone and called the office. No reply. How she longed to deliver those messages. She dreaded any more calls from the waiting ones. She waited a few minutes then rang again. Thank fortune! Her husband's response is in her ear, the messages are delivered and she goes singing up the stairs.

Ting-a-ling-ling-ling-ling-ling.

It was the telephone on the Doctor's office table and a tall young fellow was ringing it. When he got the number and asked, "Is this you, Fanny?" his face took on an expression good to see. It was Fanny, and he settled back on one elbow and asked, "What you doing, Fanny?"

"Nothing, just now. What *you* doing?"

"Something a good deal better than that."

"What is it?"

"It's talking to *you*."

"Oh!"

"Is that all you have to say about it?" his voice was growing tender.

"Now, Tom, don't go to making love to me over the 'phone."

"How can I help it, sweetheart?"

"Where are you, anyway?"

"I'm in Dr. Blank's office."

"Good gracious! is *he* there? I'll ring off—good-bye."

"Wait! Fanny—Fanny!"

Fanny was waiting, but how could a mere man know that. He rang the number again with vehemence.

"Now, Tom Laurence, I want you to quit going into people's offices and talking to me this way."

"Don't you think my way is nicer than yours—huh?"

The circumflexes were irresistible.

"Well, tell me, Tom, is Dr. Blank there?"

"No, honey. He's away in the back room busy with another patient. He can't hear."

"*Another* patient? Why, Tom, you're not *sick*, are you—huh?"

Fanny's circumflexes were quite as circumflexible as Tom's and a thrill went down the young giant's spine.

"No, but I wish I was!"

At this juncture the man who could not hear came in with a face as grave and non-committal as the Sphinx, and the young man asked through the 'phone in brisk, cheery tones, "How are you this morning?" then added in a whisper, "He's here now."

"Is he? Don't talk foolish then. Why, I'm not very well."

"What's the matter?"

"I burned my eye."

"Burned your eye! Confound it! How did you *do* it?"

"With a curling iron."

"Throw the darned thing away." He turned from the telephone and said, "Doctor, a young lady has burned her eye. I want you to go out there right away."

"Where shall I go?" asked the grave doctor.

"I guess you know," and he grinned.

"All right. I'll go pretty soon."

"Don't be too long. Charge it to me."

"Fanny," he said, turning back to the 'phone, but Fanny had gone.

And soon with a smile that had memories in it the doctor took his case and left the office, the young man at his side.

Ting-a-ling-ling-ling-ling-ling.

Mary, from the living room, heard her husband's voice:

"What is it?"

"Yes."

"They won't? O, I suppose so if nobody else will. I'll be up there in a little bit." He muttered something, took his hat and went.

When he came back, he said, "This time I had to help the dead."

"To help the dead!" exclaimed Mary.

"Yes. To help a dead woman into her coffin. Everybody was afraid to touch her."

"Why?"

"The report got out that she died of smallpox. I only saw her once and could not be sure, but to be on the safe side I insisted that every precaution be taken—hence the scare."

"But how could you lift the body without help?"

"Oh, I managed it somehow. Just the same I'd rather minister to the living," said John, to which Mary gave vigorous assent.

"Old Mr. Vintner has just been 'phoning for you in a most imperious way," announced Mary as the doctor came in at the door.

"Yes, old skinflint! The maid at his house is very sick and he's so afraid they'll have to take care of her that he's determined to send her home when she can't go. She has pneumonia. She lives miles out in the country—"

Ting-a-ling-ling-ling-ling.

"Yes."

"Now see here, Vintner. Listen to me."

"Yes, I know. But a man's got to be *human*. I tell you you can't send her out in this cold. It's outrageous to—"

"Yes, I know all that, too. But it won't be long—the crisis will come in a day or two now and—"

"Damn it! Listen. Now stop that and listen. Don't you attempt it! That girl will be to drag off if you do, I tell you—"

"All right then. That sounds more like it," and he hung up the receiver.

Mary looked up. "You are not very elegant in your discourse at times, John, but I'm glad you beat," she said.

One evening the doctor came in and walked hurriedly into the dining-room. As he was passing the telephone it rang sharply in his ear.

"What is it?" he asked, hastily putting up the receiver.

An agitated voice said, "Oh, Doctor, I've just given my little girl a teaspoonful of carbolic acid! Quick! What must I do!"

"Give her some whiskey at once; then a teaspoonful of mustard in hot water. I'll be right down," and turning he went swiftly out. When he came back an hour or two later he said: "The mother got the wrong bottle. A very few minutes would have done the work. The telephone saved the child's life. This is a glorious age in which we are living, Mary."

"And to think that some little children playing with tin cans with a string stretched between them, gave to the world its first telephone message."

"Yes, I've heard that. It may or may not be true. Now let's have supper."

"Supper awaits Mr. Non-Committal-Here-As-Ever," said Mary as she laid her arm in her husband's and they went toward the dining-room together.

One evening the doctor and Mary sat chatting with a neighbor who had dropped in.

"I want to use your 'phone a minute, please," said a voice.

"Very well," said Mary, and Mrs. X. stepped in, nodded to the trio, walked to the telephone as one quite accustomed, and rang.

"I want Dr. Brown's office," she said. In a minute came the hello.

"Is this Dr. Brown? My little boy is sick. I want you to come out to see him this evening. This is Mrs. X. Will you be right out?"

"All right. Good-bye." And she departed.

The eyes of the visitor twinkled. "Our neighbor hath need of two great blessings," she said, "a telephone and a sense of humor." Mary laughed merrily, "O, we're so used to it we paid no attention," she said, "but I suppose it did strike you as rather funny."

"It's a heap better than it used to be when we didn't have telephones," said the doctor, with the hearty laugh that had helped many a downcast man and woman to look on the bright side.

"When I was a young fellow and first hung up my shingle it was a surprising thing—the number of people who could get along without me. I used to long for some poor fellow to put his head in at the door and say he needed me. At last one dark, rainy night came the quick, importunate knock of someone after a doctor. No mistaking that knock. I opened the door and an elderly woman who lived near me, asked breathlessly, 'Mr. Blank, will you do me a great favor?'

'Certainly,' I answered promptly.

'My husband is very sick and I came to see if you would go down and ask Dr. Smithson to come and see him.' I swallowed my astonishment and wrath, put on my rubber coat and went for the doctor."

"But she had the grace to come in next day," said Mary, "and tell me in much confusion that she was greatly embarrassed and ashamed. It had not entered her head until that morning that my husband was a physician."

"You see," put in the doctor, "she had not taken me seriously; in fact had not taken me at all."

"Tell us about the old man who had you come in to see if he needed a doctor," said Mary. The doctor smiled, "*That* was when I didn't count, too," he said.

"This old fellow got sick one day and wanted to send for old Dr. Brown, but being of a thrifty turn of mind he didn't want to unless he had to. He knew me pretty well so he sent for me to come and see if he *needed* a doctor. If I thought he did he'd send for Brown. I chatted with him awhile and he felt better. Next day he sent word to me again that he wished I'd stop as I went by and I did. This kept up several days and he got better and better, and finally got well *without* any doctor, as he said."

The visitor laughed, "You doctors could unfold many a tale—"

"If the telephone would permit," said Mary, as the doctor answered the old summons, took his hat and left.

"John," said Mary one day, "I wish you would disconnect the house from the office."

"No! You're a lot of help to me," protested the doctor.

"Well, I heard someone wrangling with central today because the house answered when it was the office that was wanted." She laughed. "I know there are people who fancy the doctor's wife enjoying to the utmost her 'sweet privilege' of answering the 'phone in her husband's absence. Poor, innocent souls! If they could only know the deadly weariness of it all—but they can't."

"Why, I didn't know you felt quite that way about it, Mary. I suppose I can disconnect it but—"

"But you don't see how you can? Never mind, then. We'll go on, and some sweet day you'll retire from practice. Then hully-gee! won't I be free! You didn't choose the right sort of helpmeet, John. You surely could have selected one who would enjoy thrusting herself into the reluctant confidences of people far more than this one."

"I'm resigned to my lot," laughed John, as he kissed his wife and departed.

Ting-a-ling-ling-ling. Ting-a-ling-ling-ling.

"Is this you, Doctor?"

"Yes."

"What am I ever to do with Jane?"

"Keep her in bed! That's what to do with her."

"Well, I've got a mighty hard job. She's feeling so much better, she just *will* get up."

"Keep her down for awhile yet."

"Well, maybe I can today, but I won't answer for tomorrow. She says she feels like she can jump over the house."

"She can't, though."

Laughter. "I'll do the best I can, Doctor, but that won't be much. Keeping her in bed is easier said than done," and the doctor grinned a very ready assent as he hung up the receiver.

The doctor's family was seated at dinner. Ting-a-ling-ling-ling. John rose, napkin in hand, and went while the clatter of knives and forks instantly ceased.

"Yes."

"Why didn't you do as I told you, yesterday?"

"I *told* you what to do."

"Well, did you put them in hot water?"

"Then do it. Do it right away. Have the water *hot*, now."

He came back and went on with his dinner. Mary admitted to herself a little curiosity as to what was to be put into hot water. In a few minutes the dinner was finished and the doctor was gone.

"I bet I know what that was," spoke up the small boy.

"What?" asked his sister.

"Diphtheria clothes. There's a family in town that's got the diphtheria."

Mary was relieved—not that there should be diphtheria in town, but that the answer for which her mind was vaguely groping had probably been found.

Ting-a-ling-ling-ling. When the doctor had answered the summons he told Mary he would have to go down to a little house at the edge of town about a mile away. When he came back an hour later he sat down before the fire with his wife. "I remember a night nineteen years ago when I was called to that house—a little boy was born. I used to see the little fellow occasionally as he grew up and pity him because he had no show at all. Tonight I saw him, a great strapping fellow with a good position and no bad habits. He'll make it all right now."

The doctor paused for a moment, then went on. "They didn't pay me then. I remember that. I mentioned it tonight in the young fellow's presence."

"John, you surely didn't!"

"Yes, I did. His mother said she guessed Jake could pay the bill himself."

Mary looked at this husband of hers with a quizzical smile.

"Doesn't it strike you that you are going pretty far back for your bill?"

"There's no good reason why this boy should not pay the bill if he wants to."

"No, I suppose not. But I don't believe he was so keen to get into the world as all that."

"Well, it wouldn't surprise me much if that young fellow should come into my office one of these days and offer to settle that old score now that he knows about it."

"Don't you take it if he does!" and Mary left the room quite unconscious that her pronoun was without an antecedent.

Ting-a-ling-ling-ling-ling-ling.

"Is this you, Doctor?"

"It is."

"I expect you will have to come out to our house."

"Who is it?"

"This is Mary Milton."

"What's the matter out there, Mrs. Milton?"

"Polly's gone and hurt her shoulder. I guess she run it into the ground."

"Was she thrown from a horse or a vehicle?"

"No."

"Then how could she run it into the ground?"

"Polly Milton can run *everything* into the ground!" and the tone was exasperation itself. "I come purty near havin' to send for you yesterday, but I managed to get 'er out."

"Out of *what?*"

"The clothes-wringer. She caught her stomach fast between the rollers and nearly took a piece out of it. Nobody wanted her to turn it but she would do it."

"Well, what has she done *today?*" asked the doctor, getting impatient.

"I'm plum ashamed to tell ye. She was a-playin' leap-frog."

"Good! I'd like to play it myself once more."

"I thought you'd be scandalized. Some of the girls come over to see 'er and the first thing I knowed they was out in the yard playin' leap-frog like a passel o' boys."

"That's good for 'em," announced the doctor.

"It wasn't very good for Polly."

"The shoulder is probably dislocated. I'll be out in a little while and we'll soon fix it."

"But a great big girl nearly fourteen years old oughtn't—"

"She's all right. Don't you scold her too much." He laughed as he hung up the receiver, then ordered his horse brought round and in a few minutes was on his way to the luckless maiden.

Ting-a-ling-ling-ling—three rings.

"Is this Dr. Blank?"

"Yes."

"Can you come down to James Curtis's right away?"

"Yes—I guess so. What's the matter?"

James Curtis stated the matter and the doctor put up the receiver, went to the door and looked out.

"Gee-mi-nee! It's as dark as a stack of black cats," he said.

In a little while he was off. He had to go horseback and as the horse he usually rode was lame he took Billy who was little more than a colt. Before Mary retired she went to the door and opened it. It was fearfully dark but John had said it was only a few miles. His faithful steed could find the way if he could not. John always got through somehow. With this comforting assurance she went to bed. By and by the 'phone was ringing and she was springing up and hastening to answer it. To the hurried inquiry she replied, "He is in the country."

"How soon will he be back?"

She looked at the clock. Nearly three hours since he left home.

"I expected him before this; he will surely be here soon."

A message was left for him to come at once to a certain street and number, and Mary went back to bed. But she could not sleep. Soon she was at the 'phone again, asking central to give her the residence of James Curtis.

"Hello."

"Is this Mr. Curtis?"

"Yes, ma'am."

"Is Dr. Blank there?"

"He was, but he started home about an hour ago. He ought to be there by this time."

"Thank you," said Mary, reassured. He would be home in a little bit then and she went back to her pillow.

It was well she could not know that her husband was lost in the woods. The young horse, not well broken to the roads, had strayed from the beaten path. The doctor had first become aware of it when his hat was brushed off by low branches. He dismounted, and holding the bridle on one arm, got down on hands and knees and began feeling about with both hands in the blackness. It seemed a fruitless search, but at last he found it and put it securely on his head. He did not remount, but tried to find his way back into the path.

After awhile the colt stopped suddenly. He urged it on. Snap! A big something was hurled through the bushes and landed at the doctor's feet with a heavy thud. The pommel of the saddle had caught on a grape vine and the girths had snapped with the strain. John made a few remarks while he was picking it up and a few more while he was getting it on the back of the shying colt. But he finally landed it and managed to get it half-fastened. He stood still, not knowing which way to turn. A dog was barking somewhere—he would go in that direction. Still keeping the bridle over his arm he spread his hands before him and slowly moved on.

At last he stopped. He seemed to be getting no nearer to the dog. All at once, and not a great way off, he saw a fine sight. It was a lighted doorway with the figure of a man in it. He shouted lustily,

"Bring a lantern out here, my friend, if you please. I guess I'm lost."

"All right," the man shouted back and in a few minutes the lantern was bobbing along among the trees. "Why, Doctor!" exclaimed James Curtis, "have you been floundering around all this time in these woods so close to the house? Why didn't you holler before?"

"There didn't seem to be anything to 'holler' at. Until that door opened I thought I was in the middle of these woods."

"Your wife just telephoned to know if you were at our house and I told her you started home an hour ago."

"She'll be uneasy. Put me into the main road, will you, and we'll make tracks for home."

When he got there and had told Mary about it, she vowed she would not let him go to the country again when the night was so pitch dark, realizing as she made it, the futility of her vow. Then she told him of the message that had come in his absence and straightway sent him out again into the darkness.

It was midnight. The doctor was snoring so loudly that he had awakened Mary. Just in time. Ting-a-ling-ling-ling-ling. By hard work she got him awake. He floundered out and along toward the little tyrant. He reached it.

"Hello. What is it?"

"O! I got the wrong number."

"Damnation!"

Slumber again. After some time Mary was awakened by her husband's voice asking, "What is it?"

"It's time for George to take his medicine. We've been having a dispute about it. I said it was the powder he was to take at two o'clock and he said it was the medicine in the bottle. Now he's mad and won't take either."

"It was the powder. Tell him I say for him to take it now."

The answering voice sank to a whisper, but the words came very distinctly, "I'm afraid he won't do it—he's so stubborn. I wish it was the bottle medicine because I believe he would take that."

The doctor chuckled. "Give him that," he said. "It won't make a great deal of difference in this case, and thinking he was in the right will do him more good than the powder. Good night and report in the morning."

The report in the morning was that George was better!

It was a lovely Sabbath in May. The doctor's wife had been out on the veranda, looking about her. Everywhere was bloom and beauty, fragrance and song. Long she sat in silent contemplation of the scene. At last a drowsiness stole over her and she went in and settled herself for a doze in the big easy chair.

Soon a tinkling fell upon her drowsy ear.

"Oh! that must have been the telephone. I wonder if it was two rings or three—I'd better listen," she said with a sigh as she pulled herself up.

"Is this Dr. Blank?" The voice was faint and indistinct.

"Hello?" said Mary's husband's voice, with the rising inflection.

"Hello?" A more pronounced rise. No answer.

"Hello!" falling inflection. Here Mary interposed.

"It's some lady, Doctor, I heard her."

"Hello!" with a fiercely falling inflection.

"Dr. Blank," said the faint voice, "I forgot how you said to take those red tablets." Mary caught all the sentence though only the last three words came distinctly.

"Yes?" Her husband's 'yes' was plainly an interrogation waiting for what was to follow. She understood. He had heard only the words "those red tablets." Again she must interpose.

"Doctor, she says she forgot how you told her to take those red tablets."

"O! Why, take one every—"

Mary hung up the receiver and went back to resume her interrupted nap. She settled back on the cushions and by and by became oblivious to all about her. Sweetly she slept for awhile then started up rubbing her eyes. She went hurriedly to the 'phone and put the receiver to her ear. Silence.

"Hello?" she said. No answer. Smiling a little foolishly she went back to her chair. "It isn't surprising that I dreamed it." For a few minutes she lay looking out into the snow flakes of the cherry blooms. Then came the bell—three rings.

"I hope it's John asking me to drive to the country," she thought as she hurried to the 'phone. It was not. It was a woman's voice asking,

"How much of that gargle must I use at a time?"

"Oh dear," thought Mary, "what questions people do ask! When a gargler is a-gargling, I should think she could *tell* how much to use."

The doctor evidently thought so too for he answered with quick impatience, "Aw-enough to *gargle* with." Then he added, "If it's too strong weaken it a little."

"How much water must I put in it?" Mary sighed hopelessly and stayed to hear no more. Again she sank back in her chair hoping fervently that no more foolish questions were to rouse her from it.

When she was dozing off the bell rang so sharply she was on her feet and at the 'phone almost before she knew it.

"Doctor, the whole outfit's drunk again down here."

A woman's voice was making the announcement.

"Is that so?" The doctor's voice was calm and undisturbed.

"Yes. The woman's out here in the street just jumpin' up and down. I think *she's* about crazy."

"She hasn't far to go."

"Her father's drunk too and so's her husband. Will you come down?"

"No, I don't think I'll come down this time."

"Well, then will you send an officer?"

"No-o—I don't—"

"I wish you *would*."

"Well, I'll try to send someone."

Mary was at last too wide awake to think of dozing. This blot on the sweet May Sabbath drove away all thought of day dreams. Poor, miserable human creatures! Poor, long-suffering neighbors, and poor John!

"All sorts of people appeal to him in all sorts of cases, and often in cases which do not come within a doctor's province at all—he is guide, counsellor and friend," she thought as she put on her hat and went out for a walk.

# CHAPTER IX.

One Sunday morning at the beginning of August, Mary stood in the church—as it chanced, in the back row—and sang with her next neighbor from the same hymn book, John Newton's good old hymn,

> "Amazing grace, how sweet the sound
>
> That saved a wretch like me!"

It was the opening hymn and they were in the midst of the third verse.

> "Thro' many dangers, toils and snares,
>
> I have already come";

sang Mary.

She did not dream that another danger, toil and snare was approaching her at that instant from the rear and so her clear soprano rang out unfaltering on the next line—

> "'Tis grace that brought me safe thus far—"

Then a hand was laid upon her shoulder. She turned and started as she saw her husband's face bending to her. What had happened at home?

"Wouldn't you like to go to the country?" whispered the doctor.

"Why—I don't like to leave church to go," Mary whispered back.

"The carriage is right here at the door."

The next instant she had taken her parasol from behind the hymn-books in front of her, where she had propped it a few minutes before, with some misgiving lest it fall to the floor during prayer, and just as the congregation sang the last line,

> "And grace will lead me home,"

she glided from the church by the side of the doctor, thankful that in the bustle of sitting down the congregation would not notice her departure. They descended the steps, entered the waiting carriage and off they sped.

"I feel guilty," said Mary, a little dazed over the swift transfer. The doctor did not reply. In another minute she turned to him with energy.

"John, what possessed you to come to *the church*?"

"Why, I couldn't get you at home. I drove around there and Mollie said you had gone to church so I just drove there."

"You ought to have gone without me."

The doctor smiled. "You didn't *have* to go. But you are better off out here than sitting in the church." The horse switched his tail over the reins and the doctor, failing in his effort to release them, gave vent to a vigorous expletive.

"Yes, I certainly do hear some things out here that I wouldn't be apt to hear in there," she said. Then the reins being released and serenity restored, they went on.

"Isn't that a pretty sight?" The doctor nodded his head toward two little girls in fresh white dresses who stood on the side-walk anxiously watching his approach. There was earnest interest in the blue eyes and the black. Near the little girls stood a white-headed toddler of about two years and by his side a boy seven or eight years old.

"Mr. Blank," called the blue-eyed little girl—all men with or without titles are *Mr.* to little folks;—the doctor stopped his horse.

"Well, what is it, Mamie?"

"I want you to bring my mamma a baby."

"You do!"

"Yes, sir, a boy baby. Mamie and me wants a little brother," chimed in the little black-eyed girl.

The boy looked down at the toddler beside him and then at the two little girls with weary contempt. "You don't know what you're a-gittin' into," he said. "If this one hadn't never learned to walk it wouldn't be so bad, but he jist learns *everything* and he jist bothers me *all the time*."

The doctor and Mary laughed with great enjoyment. "Now! what'd I tell you!" said the boy, as he ran to pick up the toddler who at that instant fell off the sidewalk. He gave him a vigorous shake as he set him on his feet and a roar went up. "Don't you *git* any baby at your house," he said, warningly.

"Yes, bring us one, Mr. Blank, please do, a little *bit* of a one," said Mamie, and the black eyes pleaded too.

"Well, I'll tell you. If you'll be good and do whatever your mamma tells you, maybe I *will* find a baby one of these days and if I do I'll bring it to your house." He drove on.

"If they knew what I know their little hearts would almost burst for joy. Their father is just as anxious for a boy as they are, too," he added.

They were soon out in the open country. It was one of those lovely days which sometimes come at this season of the year which seem to belong to early autumn; neither too warm nor too cool for comfort. A soft haze lay upon the landscape and over all the Sunday calm. They turned into a broad, dusty road. Mary's eyes wandered across the meadow on the right with its background of woods in the distance. A solitary cow stood contentedly in the shade of a solitary tree, while far above a vulture sailed on slumbrous wings.

The old rail fence and the blackberry briars hugging it here and there in clumps; small clusters of the golden-rod, even now a pale yellow, which by and by would glorify all the country lanes; the hazel bushes laden with their delightful promise for the autumn—Mary noted them all. They passed unchallenged those wayside sentinels, the tall mullein-stalks. The Venus Looking-Glass nodded its blue head ever so gently as the brown eyes fell upon it and then they went a little way ahead to where the blossoms of the elderberry were turning into tiny globules of green. Mary asked the doctor if he thought the corn in the field would ever straighten up again. A wind storm had passed over it and many of the large stalks were almost flat upon the earth. The doctor answered cheerfully that the sun would pull it up again if Aesop wasn't a fraud.

After a while they stopped at a big gate opening into a field.

"Hold the reins, please, till I see if I can get the combination of that gate," and the doctor got out. Mary took a rein in each hand as he opened the gate. She clucked to the horse and he started.

"Whoa! John, come and get my mite. It's about to slip out of my glove." The doctor glanced at the coin Mary deposited in his palm.

"They didn't lose much."

"The universal collection coin, my dear. Now open the gate wider and I'll drive through."

"Don't hit the gate post!" She looked at him with disdain. "I never drove through a gate in my life that somebody didn't yell, 'Don't hit the gate post' and yet I never *have* hit a gate post."

At this retort the doctor had much ado to get the gate fastened and pull himself into the buggy, and his laughter had hardly subsided before they drew up to the large farm house in the field. Mary did not go in. In about twenty minutes the doctor came out. The door-step turned, almost causing him to fall. "Here's a fine chance for a broken bone and some of you will get it if you don't fix this step," he growled.

"I'll fix that tomorrow," said the farmer, "but I should think you'd be the last one to complain about it, Doctor."

"Some people seem to think that doctors and their wives are filled with mercenary malice," said Mary laughing. "Yesterday I was walking along with a lady when I stopped to remove a banana skin from the sidewalk. She said she would think a doctor's wife wouldn't take the trouble to remove banana skins from the walk."

"I believe in preventive medicine," said the doctor, "and mending broken steps and removing banana peeling belong to it."

"Do you think it will ever be an established fact?" asked Mary as they drove away.

"I do indeed. It will be the medicine of the future."

"I'm glad I'm not a woman of the future, then, for I really don't want to starve to death."

"I have to visit a patient a few miles farther on," said the doctor when they came out on the highway. Soon they were driving across a knoll and fields of tasseled corn lay before them. A little farther and they entered the woods. "Ah, Mary, I would not worry about leaving church. The groves were God's first temples." After a little he said, "I was trying to think what Beecher said about trees—it was something like this: 'Without doubt better trees there might be than even the most noble and beautiful now. Perhaps God has in his thoughts much better ones than he has ever planted on this globe. They are reserved for the glorious land.'"

"See this, John!" and Mary pointed to a group of trees they were passing, "a ring cut around every one of them!"

"Yes, the fool's idea of things is to go out and kill a tree by the roadside—often standing where it can't possibly do any harm. How often in my drives I have seen this and it always makes me mad."

They drove for a while in silence, then Mary said, "Nature seems partial to gold." She had been noting the Spanish needles and Black-eyed Susans which starred the dusty roadside and filled the field on the left with purest yellow, while golden-rod and wild sunflowers bloomed profusely on all sides.

"Yes, that seems to be the prevailing color in the wild-flowers of this region."

"That reminds me of something. A few months ago a little girl said to me, 'Mrs. Blank, don't you think red is God's favorite color?' 'Why, dear, I don't think I ever thought about it,' I answered, quite surprised. 'Well, I think he likes *red* better than any color.' 'Why I don't know, but when we look around and see the grass and the trees and the vines growing everywhere, it seems to me that *green* might be his favorite color. But what makes you think it is red?' 'Because he put *blood* into everybody in the world.' Quite staggered by this reasoning and making an effort to keep from smiling, I said, 'But we can't see that. If red is his favorite color why should he put it where it can't be seen?' The child looked at me in amazement. '*God* can see it. He can see clear *through* anybody.' The little reasoner had vanquished me and I fled the field."

A little way ahead lay a large snake stretched out across the road.

"The boy that put it there couldn't help it," said the doctor, "it's born in him. When I was a lad every snake I killed was promptly brought to the road and stretched across it to scare the passers-by."

"And yet I don't suppose it ever did scare anyone."

"Occasionally a girl or woman uttered a shriek and I felt repaid. I remember one big girl walking along barefooted; before she knew it she had set her foot on the cold, slimy thing. The way she yelled and made the dust fly filled my soul with a frenzy of delight. I rolled over and over in the weeds by the roadside and yelled too."

A sudden turn in the road brought the doctor and his wife face to face with a young man and his sweetheart. Mary knew at a glance they were sweethearts. They were emerging into the highway from a grassy woods-road which led down to a little church. The young man was leading two saddled horses.

"Why do you suppose they walk instead of riding?" asked the doctor.

"Hush! they'll hear you. Isn't she pretty?"

The young man assisted his companion to her seat in the saddle. She started off in one direction, while he sprang on his horse and galloped away in the other. "Here! you rascal," the doctor called, as he passed, "why didn't you go all the way with her?"

"I'll go back tonight," the young fellow called back, dashing on at so mad a pace that the broad rim of his hat stood straight up.

"Do you know him?"

"I know them both."

After another mile our travelers went down one long hill and up another and stopped at a house on the hilltop where lived the patient. Here, too, Mary chose to remain in the buggy. A wagon had stopped before a big gate opening into the barnyard and an old man in it was evidently waiting for someone. He looked at Mary and she looked at him; but he did not speak and just as she was about to say good morning, he turned and looked in another direction. When he finally looked around it seemed to Mary it would be a little awkward to bid him good morning now, so she tried to think what to say instead, by way of friendly greeting; it would be a little embarrassing to sit facing a human being for some time with not a word to break the constraint. But the more she cudgeled her brain the farther away flew every idea. She might ask him if he thought we were going to have a good corn crop, but it was so evident that we were, since the crop was already made that that remark seemed inane. The silence was beginning to be oppressive. Her eye wandered over the yard and she noticed some peach trees near the house with some of the delicious fruit hanging from the boughs. She remarked pleasantly, "I see they have some peaches here." Her companion looked at her and said, "Hey?"

"I said, 'I see they have some peaches here,'" she rejoined, raising her voice. He curved one hand around his ear and said again, "Hey?"

"O, good gracious," thought Mary, "I wish I had let him alone."

She shrieked this time, "I only said, *I see they have some peaches here.*"

When the old man said, "I didn't hear ye yet, mum," she leaned back in the carriage, fanning herself vigorously, and gave it up. She had screamed as loud as she intended to scream over so trivial a matter. Looking toward the house she saw a tall young girl coming down the walk with something in her hand. She came timidly through the little gate and handed a plate of peaches up to the lady in the carriage, looking somewhat frightened as she did so. "I didn't hear ye," she explained, "but Jim came in and said you was a-wantin' some peaches."

Mary's face was a study. Jim and his sister had not seen the deaf old man in the wagon, as a low-branched pine stood between the wagon and the house. And this was the way her politeness was interpreted!

The comicality of the situation was too much. She laughed merrily and explained things to the tall girl who seemed much relieved.

"I ought to 'a' brought a knife, but I was in such a hurry I forgot it." Eating peaches with the fuzz on was quite too much for Mary so she said, "Thank you, but we'll be starting home in a moment, I'll not have time to eat them. But I am very thirsty, might I have a glass of water?" The girl went up the walk and disappeared into the house. Mary did so want her to come out and draw the water, dripping and cool, from the old well yonder. She came out, went to the well, stooped and filled the glass from the bucket sitting inside the curb. Mary sighed. The tall girl took a step. Then, to the watcher's delight, she threw the water out, pulled the bucket up and emptied it into the trough, and one end of the creaking well-sweep started downward while the other started upward. The bucket was on its way to the cool depths and Mary grew thirstier every second.

The doctor appeared at the door and looked out. Then he came, case in hand, with swift strides down the walk. The gate banged behind him and he untied the horse in hot haste, looking savagely at his wife as he did so.

"I suppose you've asked that girl to bring you a drink."

"Yes, I did. I'm very thirsty."

"You ought to have more sense than to want to drink where people have typhoid fever."

The girl started down the walk with the brimming glass. The doctor climbed into the buggy and turned around.

"For pity's sake! what will she think?"

A vigorous cut from the whip and the horse dashed off down the road. Mary cast a longing, lingering look behind. The girl stood looking after them with open mouth.

"That girl has had enough today to astonish her out of a year's growth," thought Mary as the buggy bumped against a projecting plank and tore over the bridge at the foot of the hill.

"John, one of the rules of good driving is never to drive fast down hill." Her spouse answered never a word.

After a little he said, "I didn't mean to be cross, Mary, but I didn't want you to drink there."

"You should have warned me beforehand, then," she said chillingly.

"I couldn't sit in the buggy and *divine* there was typhoid fever there," she continued. "'A woman's intuitions are safe guides' but she has to have *something* to go on before she can *have* intuitions."

"Hadn't you better put your ulster on, dear?" inquired the doctor in such meaning tones, that Mary turned quickly and looked off across the fields. A Black-eyed Susan by the roadside caught the smile in her eyes and nodded its yellow head and smiled mischievously back at her. It was a feminine flower and they understood each other.

When they had driven three or four miles Mary asked the doctor if there was any typhoid fever in the house they were approaching.

"How do I know?"

"I thought you might be able to divine whether there is or not."

"We'll suppose there isn't. We'll stop and get a drink," he answered indulgently. They stopped, Mary took the reins and the doctor went to reconnoiter.

"Nobody at home and not a vessel of any kind in sight," he announced coming back. Of course her thirst was now raging.

"Maybe there's a gourd hanging inside the curb. If there is do break it loose and bring it to me heaping full."

"I looked inside the curb—nothing there."

Here Mary's anxious eyes saw a glass fruit jar turned upside down on a fence paling. Blessings on the woman who put it there! The doctor filled and brought it to her. After a long draught she uttered a sigh of rich content.

"Now," she said, "I'm ready to go home."

# CHAPTER X.

Ting-a-ling-ling-ling. Ting-a-ling-ling-ling.

"Hello."

"Is this the doctor?"

"It's one of 'em," said John, recognizing the voice of a patient.

"Well, doctor, the *other* side of my throat is sore *now!*"

"Is it? Well, I told your husband it might be."

"Why?"

"Why? Well, because I'm running short of coffee and a few things like that."

A little laugh. "*I* don't want to keep you in coffee and things like that."

"Nobody does. But the poor doctors have to live and you must contribute your share." Laughter.

"All right, Doctor, but I don't want to have to contribute too much."

"Don't be alarmed about your throat, Mrs. Channing. When I looked at it yesterday, I saw indications that the other side might be affected, but it will soon be well."

"That sounds better. Thank you, good-bye." When he came back to the table his wife said, "John, I shouldn't think you'd say things like that to people."

"Why?"

"Well, they might believe 'em." The doctor laughed, swallowed his cup of tea and departed.

Ting-a-ling-ling-ling. Three times.

"Hello."

"Is Dr. Blank at home?"

"He has just this minute left for the office. 'Phone him there in two minutes and you will get him."

Mary went back, took two bites and when the third was suspended on her fork the 'phone rang.

"Somebody else," she thought, laying the fork down and rising.

"Oh! I've got you again, Mrs. Blank. You said to ring in two minutes and I'd get the doctor."

"But you didn't wait *one* minute."

"It seemed lots longer. All right, I'll wait."

"People expect a doctor to get there in less than no time," thought Mary. "John walks so fast I felt safe in telling her to 'phone him in two minutes."

*Buzz-z-z-z-z,* as if all the machinery of the universe were let loose in her ear. She had held the receiver till her husband could reach the office so she might feel assured the anxious one had found him. Yes, that was his voice.

"Dr. Blank, you're president of the board of health, ain't ye?"

"Yes—guess so."

"This is Jack Johnson's. There's a dead horse down here by our house an' I want you to come down here an' bury it." Our listener heard the woman's teeth snap together.

"All right. I'll get a spade and come right along."

"What do they take my husband for," thought Mary.

Buzz-z-z-z at her ear again. Now it was her husband's voice saying,

"Give me number forty-five."

In a minute a gentlemanly voice said, "Hello."

"Is this you, Warner?"

"Yes."

"There's a dead horse down by Jack Johnson's. Go down there and bury it."

"All right, Doc. I'll be right along."

A burst of laughter from the doctor was echoed by Warner. Mary knew that Warner was the newly elected alderman and she smiled as she pictured the new officer leaving his elegant home and going down to perform the obsequies. Nevertheless her heart leaned toward Jack Johnson's wife, for it was plain to be seen that neither the new president of the board of health nor the new alderman had a realizing sense of his duties.

Half an hour later three rings sounded.

"Is this Dr. Blank's office?"

"No, his residence."

"Well, I see by the paper he's on the board of health and we want this manure-pile taken away from here."

"Please 'phone your complaints to the doctor," said Mary, calmly replacing the receiver and shutting off the flood.

"John's existence will be made miserable by this new honor thrust upon him," she thought.

When he came home that evening she asked if the second complainant had found him.

"Yes, she found me all right."

"They're going to make day hideous and night lamented, aren't they?"

"O, no. I'll just have a little fun and then send someone to look after their complaints."

Just before bed-time the doctor was called to the 'phone.

"Doctor, this is the nurse at the hotel. What had I better do with this Polish girl's hand?"

"Doesn't it look all right?"

"Yes, it's doing fine."

"Just let it alone, then."

"She won't be satisfied. She thinks we ought to be doing something to it. And I've got to do something or she'll go off upstairs and wash it in dirty water."

"Tell her not to do anything of the kind."

"She can't understand a word I say and I don't know what to do with her. She's had the bandage off once already."

"The devil she has! Well, then you'll have to unwrap it, I guess, and pretend to do something. But it would be better to let it alone."

"I know that."

"How is the other patient tonight?"

"Doing fine, Doctor."

"Good! Good-bye."

There was a spacious, airy, upper chamber opening out on a balcony at the doctor's house which the doctor and Mary claimed for theirs. Not now; O no! But in the beautiful golden sometime when the telephone ceased from troubling and the weary ones might rest. This meant when the doctor should retire from night practice. Until that happy time they occupied a smaller room on the first floor as it was near the telephone. Mary had steadfastly refused to have the privacy of her upper rooms invaded by the tyrant.

One warm summer night when bed-time came she made the announcement that she was going upstairs to sleep in the big room.

"But what if I should be called out in the night?" asked her husband, with protest in his voice.

"Then I'd be safer up there than down here," said Mary, calmly.

"But I mean you couldn't hear the 'phone."

"That is a consummation devoutly to be wished."

"Now don't go off up there," expostulated John. "You always hear it and I sort of depend on you to get me awake."

"Exactly. But it's a good thing for a man to depend on himself once in awhile. I was awake so often last night that I'm too tired and sleepy to argue. But I'm going. Good night."

"Thunder!"

"It doesn't ring *every* night," said Mary, comfortingly from the landing. "Let us retire in the fond belief that curfew will not ring tonight."

When she retired she fell at once into deep sleep. For two hours she slept sweetly on. Then she was instantly aroused. The figure of a man stood by her side. In the moonlight she saw him plainly, clad in black. Her heart was coming up into her throat when a voice said,

"Mary, I have to go two miles into the country."

"Why didn't you call me, John, instead of standing there and scaring me to death?"

"I did call you but I couldn't get you awake."

"Then you ought to have let me be. If a woman hasn't a right to a night's sleep once in awhile what *is* she entitled to?"

This petulance was unusual with his wife. "Well, come on down now, Mary," he said, kindly.

"I'm not going down there this night."

"But you can't hear the 'phone up here and I'm expecting a message any minute that must be answered."

"I'll—hear—that—'phone," said Mary. "I'll sleep with one ear and one eye open."

"Have it your own way," said the doctor as he started down the stairs.

"I intend to. But when I tell you I'll watch the 'phone, John, you know I'll do it."

He was gone and she lay wide awake. It seemed very hard to be ruthlessly pulled from a sleep so deep and delicious and so much needed.

By and by her eye-lids began to feel heavy and her thoughts went wandering into queer places. "This won't do," she said aloud, sitting up in bed. Then she rose and went out on to the balcony. Seating herself in an arm chair, she looked about her on the silvery loveliness. The cricket's chirr and the occasional affirmations of the katy-did were the only sounds she heard. "I didn't say you didn't. Don't be so spiteful about it."

The moon, shining through the branches of the big oak tree made faintly-flickering shadows at her feet. The white hammock, stirring occasionally as a breeze touched it, invited her. She went over to it and lay for many minutes looking up, noting how fast the moon glided from one branch of the tree to another. Now it neared the trunk. Now a slice was cut off its western rim. Now it was only a half moon—"a bweak-moon on the sky," as her little boy had called it. Now there was a total eclipse. When it began peeping out on the other side of the trunk our watcher's dreamful eyes took no note of it. A dog barked. She sprang up and seated herself in the chair again. She dare not trust herself to the hammock. It was too seductive and too delightful. So she sat erect and waited for the ring which might not come but which must be watched for just the same. Her promise had gone forth. Far up the street she heard horses' hoofs—it must be John returning. The buggy-top shining in the moonlight came into view. No, it was a white horse. Her vigil was not yet ended. A quarter of an hour later she discerned a figure far down the walk. She followed it with her eyes. It moved swiftly on. Would it turn at the corner and come up toward their house? Yes, it was turning. Then it turned into the yard. It was John. She went forward and leaning over the railing called down to him, "A good chance to play Romeo now, John." John only grunted—after the manner of husbands.

"Nobody rang. I'm going to bed again. Good night—I mean good morning."

The next night was hotter than ever and Mary made up her mind she would sleep up in the hammock. She had had a delicious taste of it which made her wish for more. To avoid useless discussion she would wait till John retired and was asleep, then she would quietly steal away. But when this was accomplished and she had settled herself comfortably to sleep she found herself wide awake. She closed her eyes and gently wooed slumber, but it came not. Ah, now she knew! The night before she had shaken off all responsibility for the 'phone. Therefore she could sleep. Tonight her husband lay unconscious of her absence and the burden of it was upon her shoulders again. Well, she must try to sleep anyway, this was too good a chance to lose. She fell asleep. After awhile dinner was ready. Mollie had rung the little bell for the boys. Now she was ringing it again. Where can the boys have got to? Ting-a-ling-ling-ling. Ting-a-ling-ling-ling. Ting-a-ling-ling-ling. Mary sat up in the hammock and rubbed her eyes.

"Oh!" she sprang out and rushed to the stairs. "Doctor!"

"John!" The snores continued. Ting-a-ling-ling-ling-ling-ling!

"Oh, dear!" gasped Mary, hurrying down as fast as her feet could take her. Straight to the 'phone she went. It must be appeased first.

"Hello?"

"Hell-o! Where's the doctor?"

"He is very fast asleep."

"I've found that out. Can you get him awake?" Sharp impatience was in the man's voice.

"Hold the 'phone a minute, please, and I'll rouse him."

She went into the bedroom and calling, "John! John!" shook him soundly by the shoulders. He sat up in bed with a wild look.

"Go to the 'phone, quick!" commanded Mary.

"Eh?"

"Go to the 'phone. It's been ringing like fury. Hurry."

At last he was there and his wife knew by his questions and answers that he would be out for the rest of the night. She crept into bed. After he was gone she would go upstairs. When he was dressed he came to the door and peered in.

"That's right, Mary," he said, with such hearty satisfaction in his tones that she answered cheerfully, "All right—I'll stay this time."

And when he was gone she turned her face from the moonlit window and slept till morning, oblivious to the thieves and murderers that did not come.

Ting-a-ling-ling-ling. Ting-a-ling-ling-ling.

"Is the doctor there?"

"He was called out awhile ago; will be back in perhaps twenty minutes."

"This is Mr. Cowan. I only wanted to ask if my wife could have some lemonade this morning. She is very thirsty and craves it—but I can call again after awhile."

How discouraging to the feverish, thirsty wife to have her husband come back and tell he would 'phone again after awhile. And if, after waiting, he still failed to find the doctor? Mary knew the Cowans quite well so she made bold to say, hastily, "I think the doctor would say *yes*."

"You think he would?" asked Mr. Cowan, hopefully.

"I think he would, but don't let her have too much, of course."

"All right. Thank you, Mrs. Blank."

An uneasy feeling came into Mary's mind and would not depart as she went about her work. Really, what right had she to prescribe for a sick woman even so harmless a thing as lemonade. How did she know that it was harmless. Perhaps in this case there was some combination of symptoms which would make that very thing the thing the patient ought not to have.

In about fifteen minutes there came a ring—three. Mary started guiltily. It sounded like the doctor's ring. Was he going to reprimand her? But it was the voice of a friend and it surprised Mary with this question:

"Mrs. Blank, if you were me would you have your daughter operated upon?"

"Operated upon for what?"

"For appendicitis."

"Nettie, let me tell you something: if I had no more sense than to give you advice on such a question as that, I certainly hope you would have more sense than to take it. Advice about a thing with no sort of knowledge of that thing is as worthless as it is common."

"Why—I thought since you are a doctor's wife you would know about it."

"Can you draw up a legal will because you happen to be the wife of a lawyer?"

"No-o, but—"

"But me no buts," quoth Mary. "We're even now."

"Well, I've heard it said a doctor's wife knows even less than many others about ills and their remedies because she is so used to depending on her husband that she never has to think of them herself. I guess I'd better talk to the doctor. I just thought I'd see what you said first. Good-bye."

"My skirts are clear of any advice in that direction," thought Mary, her mind reverting again to the lemonade.

"Nettie couldn't have 'phoned me at a more opportune minute to get the right answer. But I wonder if John is back. I'll see." She rang.

"Hello."

"Say, John, Mr. Cowan 'phoned awhile ago, and his wife was very thirsty and craved lemonade and—don't scold—I took the liberty of saying—it's awful for a thirsty person to have to wait and wait you know—and so I said I thought *you* would say she might have it."

"I hope you weren't this long about it," laughed her husband.

"Then it was all right?"

"Certainly." Much relieved Mary hung up the receiver. "What needless apprehension assails us sometimes," she thought, as she went singing to her broom.

"Just the same, I won't prescribe very often."

# CHAPTER XI.

It was five o'clock in the morning when the doctor heard the call and made his way to it. His wife was roused too and was a passive listener.

"Yes."

"Yes."

"Down where? I don't understand you."

"On what street?.... Down near Dyre's? I don't know any such family." Here Mary called out, "Maybe they mean Dye's."

"Dye's? Yes, I know where that is..... Galliver—that's the name is it? Very well, Mrs. Galliver, I'll be down in a little while.... Yes, just as soon as I can dress and get there."

He proceeded to clothe himself very deliberately, but years of repression had taught Mary resignation.

Ting-a-ling-ling-ling. Three rings.

The doctor went with shoe in hand and again his wife was a listener.

"Yes..... Yes..... I'm just getting ready to go to see a patient...... It's a hurry call, is it? All right then, I'll come there first...... Yes, right away."

As he put up the receiver he said to his wife, "Somebody else was trying to get me then, too, but couldn't make it." Mary thought it well he couldn't since her husband was only one and indivisible.

"But he will probably try again after a little," she thought, "and John will be gone and I won't know just where to find him."

Ting-a-ling-ling-ling-ling-ling. Collar in hand the doctor went.

"Yes..... Who is this?.... Come where?.... Jackson street. Right next to Wilson's mill?.... On which side? I say on which side of Wilson's mill?.... West? All right, I'll be down there after awhile...... No, not right away; I have to make two other visits first, but as soon as I can get there."

When at last he was dressed and his hand was on the door-knob the 'phone called him back.

"You say I needn't come..... Very well. I'll come if you want me to though, Mrs. Galliver. I'm just starting now. I have to see another patient first."—

"Why John," interposed Mary from the bedroom, "She called you first."

"It will be about half an hour before I can get there..... All right, I'll be there."

Then Mary remembered that No. 2 was the hurry call and was silent. When the doctor was gone she fell asleep but only for two minutes.

She went to answer the call. "Has the doctor started yet?"

"Yes, he is on his way."

"All right then," and the relief in the tone was a pleasant thing to hear.

"Now, if I go to sleep again I can feel no security from No. 1 or No. 3 or both." Nevertheless she did go to sleep and neither No. 1 nor No. 3 called her out of it.

"I must be going," said Mary, rising from her chair in a neighbor's house.

"Have you something special on hand?" asked her neighbor.

"Yes, it's clock-winding day at our house, for one thing."

"Why, how many clocks do you have to wind?" inquired the little old lady with mild surprise.

"Only one, thank heaven!" ejaculated Mary as she departed.

When she had sped across the yard and entered her own door she threw off her shawl and made ready to wind the clock. First, she turned off the gas in the grate so that her skirts would not catch fire. Second, she brought a chair and set it on the hearth in front of the grate. Third, she went into the next room and got the big unabridged dictionary, brought it out and put it on the chair. Fourth, she went back and got the oldest and thickest Family Bible and the fat Bible Dictionary, brought them out and deposited them on the unabridged. Fifth, she mounted the chair. Sixth, she mounted the volumes—which brought her up to the height she was seeking to attain. Seventh, she wound the clock; that is, she usually did. Today, when she had inserted the key and turned it twice round—the 'phone rang. Oh, dear! Thank goodness it stopped at two rings. She would take it for granted the doctor was in the office. She wound on. Then she took the key out and inserted it on the opposite side. A second peal. That settled it. If it were a lawyer's or a merchant's or any other man's 'phone she could wind the other side first—but the doctor's is in the imperative mood and the present tense. She must descend. Slowly and cautiously she did so, went to the 'phone and put the receiver to her ear.

"Hello, is this Dr. Blank's office?"

"This is his—"

"Hello, what is it?" said her husband's voice. "Now why couldn't he have come a minute sooner," thought Mary, provoked.

"Doctor," said an agitated voice, "my little boy has swallowed a penny."

"Was it a good one?" inquired the doctor, calmly.

"Why—ye-es," said the voice, broken with a laugh, "guess it was."

"Just let him alone. It will be all right after awhile."

"It was worth getting down to hear so comforting an assurance," said Mary as she ascended again the chair and the volumes. She finished her weekly task, then slowly and cautiously descended, carried the big books back to their places, set the chair in its corner and lighted the gas. She stood for a moment looking up at this clock. The space over the mantel-piece was just the place for it and it was only after it had been firmly anchored to the wall that the thought had arisen, "How can I ever get up there to wind it?"

She smiled as she thought of a social gathering a few days before, when a lady had called to her across the room, "Mrs. Blank, tell us that clock story again." And she had answered:

"It isn't much of a story, but it serves to show the manner in which we computed the time. One night the doctor woke me up. 'Mary,' he said in a helpless sort of way, 'It struck *seven*—what *time* is it?' 'Well—let me see,' I said. 'If it struck seven it meant to strike three, for it strikes four ahead of time. And if it meant to strike three it's just a quarter past two, for it's three quarters of an hour too fast.'" Ting-a-ling-ling. Ting-a-ling-ling-ling. Ting-a-ling-ling-ling.

Mary recognized her husband's ring. "Yes, what is it John?"

"I'm going out for twenty minutes, watch the 'phone, please."

She laughed in answer to this most superfluous request, then sat her down near by.

"John, Mrs. B. said a pretty good thing last night."

"That's good."

"I've a notion not to tell you, now that the good thing was about you."

"That's better still. But are good things about me so rare that you made a note of it?"

"I don't know but what they are," said Mary, reflectively. "There was Mrs. C., you know, who said she didn't see how in the world Doc Blank's wife ever lived with him—he was so mean."

"I wonder about that myself, sometimes."

"The way I manage it is to assert myself when it becomes necessary—and it does. You're a physician to your patients but to me you're a mere man."

"I feel myself shrivelling. But how about Mrs. B.'s compliment?"

"I was over at the church where a social program of some sort was being given and 'between acts' everybody was moving about chatting. An elderly woman near me asked, 'Mrs. Blank, do you know who the Hammell's are?' I told her that I did not, and she went on, 'I see by the paper that a member of their family died today, and I thought you, being a doctor's wife, might know something about it.'

"Mrs. B. spoke up promptly, 'Why, Mrs. Blank wouldn't know anything about the *dead* people—her husband gets 'em *well*.'"

The doctor laughed, "And she believes it too," he said.

"No doubt of it. So a compliment like that offsets one of Mrs. C.'s kind."

"O, no. The C.'s have it by a big majority. Don't you know I have the reputation of being the meanest man in the county?"

"No, I don't."

"Well, I have. Do you remember that drive we took a week or two ago up north?"

"That long drive?"

"Yes. When I went in the man who was a stranger to me, said, 'I'll tell you why I sent for you. I've had two or three doctors out here, recommended as *good* doctors, and they haven't done me a darned bit of good. Yesterday I heard you was the meanest doctor in this county and I said to myself, "He's the man I want."'"

"I heard you laughing and wondered what it was about. The man's wife came out to the buggy and talked to me. She said they were strangers and didn't know anything about the doctors around here—they had thought of sending down to this town for a doctor but she had spoken to a woman—a neighbor—and she had said there wasn't *any* of 'em any account down there. But her husband kept getting worse so they finally sent for Dr. Blank and she hoped he'd cure 'im. Are you doing it? I hope so for I assured her that the physicians of this town are recognized throughout the State as being men of exceptional ability, and she went in, comforted."

"Yes, he got better as soon as he struck the road to health," laughed John. He took out his watch. "Jove! I haven't any time to spare if I catch that train." For several days he had been taking the train to a little station some miles out of town, where he would get off and walk a mile to the home of his patient, make his visit and walk back in time to catch the train for home.

Just after the doctor left the house the telephone rang twice. His wife answered it, knowing he had not yet reached the office.

"Is the doctor there?"

"He left the house just a minute ago."

"Well, he's coming down today isn't he?"

"Is this Mrs. Shortridge?"

"Yes."

"Yes, he just said he must make that train."

"He'll go to the office first won't he?"

"Yes, to get his case, I think."

"Will you please telephone him there to bring a roast with him?"

"To bring what?"

"A roast."

Mary was nonplussed. Her husband had the reputation of "roasting" his patients and their attendants on occasion. Had an occasion arisen now?

"Why, ye-es," she began, uncertainly, when the voice spoke again.

"I mean a roast of beef, Mrs. Blank. I thought as the doctor was coming he wouldn't mind stopping at the butcher's and bringing me a roast—tell him a good-sized one."

The receiver clicked. Mary still held hers. Then she rang the office.

"What *is* it?" Great haste spoke in the voice.

"John, Mrs. Shortridge wants you to bring her a roast of beef when you go down."

"The devil she does!"

"The market is right on your way. Hurry. Don't miss the train!" She put up the receiver, then she snatched it and rang again violently.

"*Now* what!" thundered John's voice.

"She said to get a good-sized one." Standing with the receiver in her hand and shaking with laughter she heard the office-door shut with a bang and knew that he was off.

She knew that if he had been going in the buggy he would have been glad to do Mrs. S.'s bidding. He often carried ice and other needful things to homes where he visited. Mary pictured her husband picking his way along a muddy country road, his case in one hand and the "roast" in the other, and thought within herself, "He'll be in a better mood for a roast when he arrives than when he started."

Mary was out in the kitchen making jelly. At the critical moment when the beaded bubbles were "winking at the brim" came the ring. She lifted the kettle to one side, wiped her hands and went.

"Is this you, Mary?"

"Yes."

"Watch the 'phone a little bit, please. I have to be out about half an hour."

"I'm always watching the 'phone, John, always, *always!*"

She went back to her jelly. She put it back on the fire, an inert mass with all the bubbles died out of it. Scarcely had she done so when the 'phone rang—two rings. Surely the doctor had not got beyond hearing distance. He would answer. But perhaps he had—he was a very swift walker. The only way to be sure of it was to go to the telephone and listen. She went hastily back and as she put the receiver to her ear there came a buzz against it which made her jump.

"Hello," she said.

"I wanted the doctor, Mrs. Blank, do you know where he is?"

"He just 'phoned me that he—" an unmistakable sound arose from the kitchen stove. The jelly was boiling over! Instinct is older than the telephone. The receiver dangled in air while Mary rushed madly to the rescue. "I might have known it," she said to herself, as she pushed the kettle aside and rushed back to the 'phone.

"I guess they cut us off," said the voice.

"I was just saying," said Mary, "that the doctor 'phoned me a few minutes ago he would be out for half an hour."

"Will you please tell him when he comes in to call up 83?"

The man goes on his way, relieved of further responsibility in the matter. It will be a very easy thing for the doctor's wife to call up her husband and give him the message. Let us see.

When the jelly was done, and Mary had begun to fill the waiting glasses she thought, "I'd better see if John is back. He may go out again before I can deliver that message." So she set the kettle on the back of the stove and went to ascertain if her husband had returned. No answer to her ring. She had better ring again to be sure of it. No answer. She went back to the kitchen. When the glasses were all filled and she had held first one and then another up to get the sunlight through the clear beautiful redness of them, she began setting them back to cool. The telephone! She hurried in and rang again to see if John had got back. Silence. She sighed and hung up the receiver. "I'd like to get it off my mind." As she started toward the kitchen again the door-bell rang. She went to open the door, and wonder of wonders—an old friend she had not seen for years!

"I am passing through town, Mary, and have just three quarters of an hour till my train goes. Now sit down and *talk*."

And the pair of them did talk, oblivious to everything about them. How the minutes did fly and the questions too! The 'phone rang in the next room— two rings. On Mary's accustomed ear it fell unheeded. She talked on. Again two rings. She did not notice.

"Isn't that your 'phone?" asked the visitor.

"O, *yes*! You knocked it clean out of my head, Alice. Excuse me a minute," and she vanished.

"Did you give that message to the doctor?"

"He is not back yet."

"I saw him go into the office not ten minutes ago."

"I have 'phoned twice and failed to find him."

"I hoped when I saw him leave the office that he had started down to see my little boy, but of course he hasn't if he didn't get the message."

"I am sorry. An old friend I had not seen for years came in and of course it went out of my mind for a few minutes, though I 'phoned twice before she came. I am sure he will be back in a few minutes and I will send him right down, Mr. Nelson."

"Why do you do that?" asked her friend, pointedly as she came in. "Why take upon yourself the responsibility of people's messages being delivered."

"It *is* an awful responsibility. I don't know why I do it—so many people seem to expect it as a matter of course—"

"It's a great deal easier for each person to deliver his own message than for you to have a half dozen on your mind at once. I wouldn't do it. You'll be a raving lunatic by the next time I see you."

"At least I'll have ample time in which to become one," laughed Mary.

"I'm going," announced her friend, suddenly rising. "I could spare five or ten minutes more but if I sit here you'll forget that 'phone again. But take my advice, Mary, and institute a change in the order of things."

When she had gone Mary sat for a few minutes lost in thought. Then, remembering, she sprang up and went to the 'phone. No answer to her ring. "Dear me! Will I *never* get that message delivered and off my mind." Soon a ring came.

"Isn't he back *yet?*"

"I 'phoned about three minutes ago and failed to get him. By the way, Mr. Nelson, will you just 'phone the doctor at the office, please? That will be a more direct way to get him as I seem to fail altogether this morning. I am sure that he can't be gone much longer," she said very pleasantly and hung up the receiver. The responsibility had been gracefully shifted and she was free for a while. Other occasions would arise when she could not be free, but in cases of this kind her friend's clear insight had helped her out.

Ting-a-ling-ling-ling. Ting-a-ling-ling-ling.

"Hello."

"Is this Dr. Blank?"

"Yes."

"My husband has just started for your office. He says he's going to send you down. I don't need a doctor. Will you tell him that?"

"I'll tell him you *said* so."

"Well, I don't. So don't you come!"

"All right. I haven't got time to be bothered with you anyway. The sick people take my time."

In a few minutes the 'phone rang again.

"Dr. Blank, can you come over to the Woolson Hotel?"

"Right away?"

"Yes, if you can. There's a case here I've treated a little that I'm not satisfied about."

"All right, Doctor, I'll be there in a few minutes."

When he reached the hotel and had examined the patient he said, "He has smallpox."

"I began to suspect that."

"Not a bit of doubt of it."

"The hotel is full of people—I'm afraid there'll be a panic."

"We must get him out of here. We'll have to improvise a pest-house at once. I'll go and see about it."

That evening about an hour after supper the doctor's daughter came hurriedly into the room where her mother was sitting.

"Mother," she exclaimed, "there's an awful lot of people in the office, a regular mob and they're as mad as fury."

"What about?" exclaimed her mother, startled.

"They're mad at father for putting the tent for a smallpox patient down in their neighborhood."

"Is he in the office now?"

"He was there when I first went in but he isn't there just now. Father wasn't a bit disturbed, but I am. I got out of there. The mayor went into the office just as I came out."

Uneasy, in spite of herself, Mary waited her husband's return. Ten o'clock, and he had not come. She went to the 'phone and called the office. The office man answered.

"Where is the doctor?"

"He was in here a few minutes ago, but there's a big fuss down at the smallpox tent and I think he's gone down there."

Mary rang off and with nervous haste called the mayor's residence.

"Is this Mr. Felton?"

"Yes."

"This is Mrs. Blank. I am very uneasy about the doctor, Mr. Felton. I hear he has just started down to the smallpox tent. Won't you please see that someone goes down at once?"

"Yes, Mrs. Blank. I came from there a little while ago but they're mad at the doctor and I'll go right back. I'm not going to bed until I know everything's quieted down."

"And you'll take others with you?" she pleaded, but the mayor was gone. Again she waited in great anxiety. The tent was too far away for her to go out into the night in search of him.

Between eleven and twelve o'clock she heard footsteps. She rose and went to the door. Almost she expected to see her husband brought home on a stretcher. But there he came, walking with buoyant step. When he came in he kissed his anxious wife and then broke into a laugh.

"My! how good that sounds! I heard of the mob and have been frightened out of my wits."

"They've quieted down now. There wasn't a bit of sense in what they did."

"Well, I don't know that one can really blame them for not wanting smallpox brought into the neighborhood. Couldn't you have taken the tent farther out?"

"Yes, if we had had time. But we had a sick man on our hands—he had to be got out of the hotel and he had to be taken care of right away. He had to have a nurse. There must be water in the tent and the nurse can't be running out of a pest-house to get it. Neither can anyone carry it to such a place. So we couldn't put it beyond the water- and gas-pipes—there must be heat, too, you know. We have done the very best we could without more time. The nearest house is fifty yards away and there's absolutely no danger if the people down there will just get vaccinated and then keep away from the tent."

"They surely will do that."

"Some of them may. One fool said to me awhile ago when I told them that, 'Oh, yes! we see your game. You want to get a lot of money out of us.'"

"What did you say to that ancient charge," asked Mary, smiling.

"I said, 'My man, I'll pay for the virus, and I'll vaccinate everyone of you, and everyone in that neighborhood and it won't cost you a cent'."

"Did he look ashamed?"

"I didn't wait to see. I had urgent business out just then."

"Is the patient in the tent now?"

"Yes, all snug and comfortable with a nurse to take care of him. That was my urgent business. I went into the back room of the office in the midst of their jabber, slipped out the door, got into the buggy hitched back there, drove to the hotel and with Dr. Collins' help, got the patient down the ladder waiting for us, into the buggy, then got the nurse down the ladder and in, too, then away we drove lickety-cut for the tent while the mob was away from there. Then I went back to the office and attended the meeting," added the doctor, laughing heartily.

His wife laughed too, but rather uneasily. "Were they still there when you got back?"

"Every mother's son of 'em. They didn't stay long though. I advised them to go home, that the patient was in the tent and would stay there. They broke for the tent—vowed they'd set fire to it with him in it and I think they intended to hang *me*," and the doctor laughed again.

"John, don't *ever* get into such a scrape again. I 'phoned Mr. Felton and begged him to go down there and take someone with him."

"You did? Well, he came, and it happened there was a member of the State Board of Health in town who had got on to the racket. He came, too, and you ought to have heard him read the riot act to those fellows:

"'We've got a sick man here—a stranger, far from his home. You are in no danger whatever. Every doctor in town has told you so. We're going to take care of this man *and don't you forget it*. We have the whole State of Illinois behind us, and if this damned foolishness don't stop right here, I'll have the militia here in a few hours' time and arrest every one of you.' That quieted them. They slunk off home and won't bother us any more."

Three or four days after the above conversation Mary stood at the window looking out at the storm which was raging. The wind was blowing fearfully and the rain coming down in torrents. "I do hope John will not be called to the country today," she thought.

Ting-a-ling-ling-ling—three rings.

"Is this Dr. Blank's office?" asked a feminine voice.

"No, his residence."

"Mrs. Blank, this is the nurse at the smallpox tent. Will you 'phone the office and tell the doctor it's raining in down here terribly. I'm in a hurry, must spread things over the patient."

"Very well, I'll 'phone him," and she rang twice. No reply. Again. No reply. "Too bad he isn't in. I'll have to wait a few minutes."

In five minutes she rang again, but got no reply. In another minute she was called to the 'phone.

"Didn't you get word to the doctor, Mrs. Blank?" asked a voice, full of anxiety. "I'm afraid we'll drown before he gets here."

"I have been anxiously watching for him, but he must be visiting a patient. Hold the 'phone please till I ring again." This time her husband answered.

"Doctor, here's the nurse at the tent to speak to you." She waited to hear what he would say.

"Doctor, please come down here and help us. The roof is leaking awfully and we are about to drown."

"All right, I'll be down after a little."

"Don't wait too long."

Mary's practised ear caught something beginning with a capital D as the receiver clicked.

"Poor old John," she murmured, "it's awful—the things you have to do."

The doctor got into his rubber coat and set out for his improvised pesthouse.

When he came home Mary asked, "Did you stop the leak?"

"I did. But I had a devil of a time doing it."

"I'm curious to know how you would go about it."

"The roof was double and I had to straighten out and stretch the upper canvas with the wind blowing it out of my hands and nobody to help me hold it."

"Was there nobody in sight?"

"That infernal coward of a watchman, but I couldn't get him near the tent—he's *had* smallpox, too."

"I should think the nurse could have helped a little, that is if she knew where to take hold of it, and what to do with it when she got hold."

"O, she sputtered around some and imagined she was helping."

"Poor thing," said Mary, laughing, "I know just how bewildered she was with you storming commands at her which she couldn't understand—women can't."

Ting-a-ling-ling-ling. Ting-a-ling-ling-ling. Ting-a-ling-ling-ling.

The doctor helloed gruffly.

"Is this you, Doc?"

"Looks like it."

"We want ye to come down here an' diagnosis these cases."

"*What* cases!"

"There's two down here."

"Down *where?*"

"Down here at my house."

"Well, who the devil *are* you?"

"Bill Masters. We're afraid maybe it's smallpox."

"Yes, *yes!*" snarled the doctor, "every *pimple* around here for the next three months will be smallpox."

"Well, we want ye to diagnosis it, Doc."

"All right. I'll 'diagnosis' it the first time I'm down that way—maybe this evening or tomorrow," and he slammed the receiver up and went to bed.

One evening the doctor was waiting for the stork at a farmhouse some miles from home. He concluded to telephone his wife as it might be several hours before he got in. He rang and put the receiver to his ear:

"Did you put your washin' out today?"

"No, did you?"

"No, I thought it looked too rainy."

"So did I. I hope it'll clear up by mornin'."

"Have you got your baby to sleep yet?"

"Land! yes. He goes to sleep right after supper."

"Mine's not that kind of a kid. He's wider awake than any of us this minute."

"Got your dress cut out?"

"No, maybe I'll git around to it tomorrow afternoon, if I don't have forty other things to do."

"Did ye hear about—"

Seeing no chance to get in the doctor retreated. Half an hour later he rang again. A giggle and a loud girlish voice in his ear asking, "Is this you, Nettie?"

"This is me."

"Do you know who this is?"

"Course I do."

"Bet ye don't."

"Bet I do."

"Who?"

"It's Mollie, of course."

"You've guessed it. I tried to change my voice so you wouldn't know me."

"What fer?"

"Oh, cat-fur to make kitten breeches."

Mild laughter.

"I heard that you gave Jake the mitten last night."

"Who told ye?"

"Oh, a little bird."

"Say! Who *did* tell ye?"

"You'll never, never tell if I do?"

The clock near the patiently waiting doctor struck nine quick short strokes.

"Did you hear that?" asked the first voice, startled.

"Whose clock *is* that?"

"Johnson's haven't got one like that."

"Miller's haven't neither."

"I'll tell you—it's Gray's—their clock strikes quick like that."

"Then there's somebody at their 'phone listenin'!"

"Goodness! Maybe it's Jake, just like him!"

"Jake Gray, if that's you, you're a mean eavesdroppin' sneak an' that's what I think of *you*! Good-bye, Nettie." And as the receiver slammed into its place the doctor shook with laughter.

"This seems to be my opportunity," he thought, then rang and delivered the message to his wife. Often these dialogues kept him from hearing or delivering some important message and then he fumed inwardly, but tonight he had time to spare and to laugh.

After a little the 'phone rang. "It's someone wanting you, Doctor," said the man of the house who answered it. The doctor went.

"Is this you, Doctor Blank?"

"Yes."

"I want you—"

The doctor heard no more. This was a party line and every receiver on it came down. A dozen people were listening to find out who wanted the doctor and what for. All on the line knew that Doctor Blank had been at the Gray farmhouse for hours. The message being private, there was silence. The doctor waited a minute then his wrath burst forth.

"Damn it! Hang up your receivers, all you eavesdroppers, so I can get this message!"

Click, click, click, click, and lots of people mad, but the doctor got the message.

Ting-a-ling-ling-ling.

"Is this Mrs. Blank?"

"Yes."

"I telephoned the office and couldn't get the doctor so I'll tell you what I wanted and you can tell him. His patient down here in the country, Mrs. Miller, is out of powders and she wants him to send some down by Mrs. Richards, if he can find her."

"Where is Mrs. Richards?"

"She's up there in town somewhere."

"Does she know that the powders are to be sent by her and will she call at the office?"

"No, I don't think she knows anything about it. Mrs. Miller didn't know she was out till after she left. That's all," and she was gone.

"All!" echoed Mary.

In a few minutes when she thought her husband had had time to return she went to the 'phone and told him he must go out and hunt up Mrs. Richards.

"What for?"

"Because Mrs. Miller wants you to find her and send some powders down by her."

An explosion came and Mary retired laughing and marvelling to what strange uses telephones—and doctors—are put.

# CHAPTER XII.

It was a lovely morning in late September. The sun almost shone through the film of light gray clouds which lay serenely over all the heavens. There was a golden gleam in the atmosphere,

> "And a tender touch upon everything
>
> As if Autumn remembered the days of Spring."

The doctor and his wife were keenly alive to the beauty of the day. After they had driven several miles they stopped before a little brown house. The doctor said he would like Mary to go in and she followed him into the low-ceiled room.

"Here, you youngsters, go out into the yard," said the mother of the children. "There ain't room to turn around when you all get in." They went. A baby seven or eight months old sat on the floor and stared up at Mary as she seated herself near it. Two women of the neighborhood sat solemnly near by. The doctor approached the bed on which a young woman of eighteen or twenty years was lying.

"My heart hain't beat for five minutes," she said.

"Is that so?" said the doctor, quite calm in the face of an announcement so startling. "Well, we'll have to start it up again."

"That's the first time she has spoke since yesterday morning," said one of the solemn women in a low tone to the doctor.

"It didn't hurt her to keep still. She could have spoken if she had wanted to." The two women looked at each other. "No, she couldn't speak, Doctor," said one of them.

"Oh, yes she could," replied the doctor with great nonchalance.

"I *couldn't*," said the patient with much vigor. This was just what he wanted. He examined her carefully but said not a word.

"How long do you think I'll live?" she asked after a little.

"Well, that's a hard question to answer—but you ought to be good for forty or fifty years yet."

The patient sniffed contemptuously. "Huh, I guess you don't know it all if you *are* a doctor."

"I know enough to know there's mighty little the matter with *you*." He turned to one of the women. "I would like to see her mother," he said. The mother had left the room on an errand; the woman rose and went out. There was a pause which Mary broke by asking the baby's name.

"We think we'll call her Orient."

"Why not Occident?" thought Mary, but she kept still. Not so the doctor. "*That's* no name. Give her a good sensible *name*—one she won't be ashamed of when she's a woman."

Here Mary caught sight of a red string around the baby's neck, and asked if it was a charm of some sort. The mother took hold of the string and drew up the charm. "It's a blind hog's tooth," she said simply, "to make her cut her teeth easy."

The mother of the patient came into the room. "How do you think she is, Doctor?"

"Oh, she's not so sick as you thought she was, not near."

The mother looked relieved. "She had an awful bad spell last night. Do you think she won't have any more?"

"No, she won't have any more." The look on the patient's face said plainly, "We'll see about that." It did not escape the doctor.

"But in case you should see any signs of a spell coming on, and if she gets so she can't speak again, then you must—but come into the next room," he said in a low voice.

They went into an adjoining room, the doctor taking care to leave the door ajar. Then in a voice ostensibly low enough that the patient might not hear and yet so distinct that she could hear every word, he delivered his instructions: "Now, if she has any more spells she must be blistered all the way from her neck down to the end of her spine." The mother looked terrified. "And if she gets so she can't speak again, it will be necessary to put a seton through the back of her neck."

"What *is* a seton?" faltered the woman.

"Oh, it's nothing but a big needle six or eight inches long, threaded with coarse cord. It must be drawn through the flesh and left there for a while." Then in a tone so low that only the mother could hear, he said, "Don't pay much attention to her. She'll never have those spells unless there is somebody around to see her."

He walked into the other room and took up his hat and case.

"I left some powders on the table," he said to the mother. "You may give her one just before dinner and another tonight."

"Will it make any difference if she doesn't take it till tonight?"

"Not a bit."

"Pa's gone and I didn't 'low to git any dinner today."

At this announcement Mary heard something between a sigh and a groan and turning, saw a rosy-cheeked boy in the doorway. There was a look of resigned despair on his face and Mary smiled sympathetically at him as she went out. How many lads and lassies could have sympathized with him too, having been victims to that widespread feeling among housewives that when "Pa" is gone no dinner need be got and sometimes not much supper.

As the doctor and his wife started down the walk they heard a voice say, "Ma, don't you ever send for that smart-aleck doctor agin. I won't *have* him." The doctor shook with laughter as he untied the horse.

"They won't need to send for me 'agin.' I like to get hold of a fine case of hysterics once in a while—it makes things lively."

"The treatment you prescribed was certainly heroic enough," said Mary.

They had driven about a mile, when, in passing a house a young man signaled the doctor to stop. "Mother has been bleeding at the nose a good deal," he said, coming down to the gate. "I wish you would stop and see her. She'll be glad to see you, too, Mrs. Blank."

They were met at the door by a little old woman in a rather short dress and in rather large ear-rings. Her husband, two grown daughters and three children sat and stood in the room.

"So you've been bleeding at the nose, Mrs. Haig?" said the doctor, looking at his patient who now sat down.

"Yes, sir, and it's a-gittin' me down. I've been in bed part of the day."

"It's been bleedin' off and on for two days and nights," said the husband.

"Did you try pretty hard to stop it?"

"Yes, sir, I tried everything I ever heerd tell of, and everything the neighbors wanted me to try, but it didn't do no good."

"Open the door and sit here where I can have a good light to examine your nose by," the doctor said to the patient. She brought her chair and the young man opened the door. As he did so there was a mad rush between the old man and his two daughters for the door opposite.

"Shet that door, quick!" the old man shouted, and it was instantly done. Mary looked around with frightened eyes. Had some wild beast escaped from a passing menagerie and was it coming in to devour the household? There was a swirl of ashes and sparks from the big fireplace.

"This is the blamedest house that ever was built," said Mr. Haig.

"Who built it?" queried the doctor.

"I built it myself and like a derned fool went an' put the fireplace right between these two outside doors, so if you open one an' the other happens to be open the fire and ashes just flies."

The doctor took an instrument from his pocket and proceeded with his examination.

"But there's a house back here on the hill about a mile that beats this," said the old man.

"That is a queer-looking house," said Mary. "It has no front door at all."

"No side door, neither. When a feller wants to get in *that* house there's just one of three ways: he has to go around and through the kitchen, or through a winder, or down the chimney."

"If he was little enough he might go through the cat-hole," suggested the young man, at which they all laughed.

"And what may that be?" asked the mystified Mary.

"It's a square hole cut in the bottom of the door for the cat to go in and out at. The man that owns the place said he believed in having things handy."

"Now, let me see your throat," said the doctor. The patient opened her mouth to such an amazing extent that the doctor said, "No, I will stand on the outside!" which made Mary ashamed of him, but the old couple laughed heartily. They had known this doctor a good many years.

"What have you been doing to stop the bleeding?" he asked.

"I've been a-tryin' charms and conjurin', mostly."

Mary saw that there was no smile on her face or on any other face in the room. She spoke in a sincere and matter-of-fact way. "Old Uncle Peter, down here a piece, has cured many a case of nose-bleed but he hain't 'peared to help mine."

"How does he go about it?" asked Mary.

"W'y, don't you know nothin' 'bout conjurin'?"

"Nothing at all."

"I thought you bein' a doctor's wife would know things like that."

"I don't believe my husband practises conjuring much."

"Well, Uncle Peter takes the Bible, and opens it, and says some words over it, and pretty soon the bleedin' stops."

"Which stops it, the Bible or the words?"

"W'y—both I reckon, but the words does the most of it. They're the charm and nobody knows 'em but him."

"Where did he learn them?"

"His father was a conjurer and when he died he tol' the words to Uncle Peter an' give the power to him."

"Did he come up here to conjure you?" asked the doctor.

"No, he says he can do it just as well at home."

"He can. But I think we can stop the bleeding without bothering Uncle Peter any more. I'd like a pair of scissors," he said, meaning to cut some papers for powders.

"They won't do no good. I've tried 'em."

"What do you think I want with them?"

"I 'lowed you wanted to put 'em under the piller. That'll cure nose-bleed lots of times. Maybe you don't believe it, but it's so."

"Can Uncle Peter cure other things?" asked Mary.

"He can *that*. My nephew had the chills last year and shook and shook. At last he went to Uncle Peter an' he cured *him*."

"He shot 'em," said Mr. Haig.

"Yes, he told him to take sixteen shot every mornin' for sixteen days and by the time he got through he didn't shake a bit."

"By jings! he was so heavy he couldn't," said Mr. Haig, and in the laugh that followed the doctor and his wife rose to go. A neighboring woman with a baby in her arms had come in and seated herself near the door. As he passed out the doctor stopped to inquire, "How's that sore breast? You haven't been back again."

"It's about well. William found a mole at last and when I put the skin of it on my breast it cured it. I knowed it would, but when we wanted a mole there wasn't none to be found, so I had to go and see *you* about it."

"I thought it would soon be well. Good for the mole-skin," laughed the doctor, as they took their leave.

When they had started homeward they looked at each other, the doctor with a smile in his eyes—he had encountered this sort of thing so often in his professional life that he was quite accustomed to it. But Mary's brown eyes were serious. "John," she said, "when will the reign of ignorance and superstition end?"

"When Time shall be no more, my dear."

"So it seems. Those people, while lacking education, seem to be fairly intelligent and yet their lives are dominated by things like these."

"Yes, and not only people of fair intelligence but of fair education too. While they would laugh at what we saw and heard back there they are holding fast to things equally senseless and ridiculous. Then there are thoroughly educated and cultured people holding fast to little superstitions which had their birth in ignorance away back in the past somewhere. How many people do you know who want to see the new moon over the left shoulder? And didn't I hear you commanding Jack just the other day to take the hoe right out of the house and to go out the same door he came in?"

"O, ye-es, but then *nobody* wants to have a *hoe* carried through the house, John. It's such a bad sign—"

The doctor laughed. "This thing is so widespread there seems to be no hope of eliminating it entirely though I believe physicians are doing more than anybody else toward crushing it out."

"Can they reason and argue people out of these things?"

"Not often. Good-natured ridicule is an effective shaft and one I like to turn upon them sometimes. They get so they don't want to say those things to me, and so perhaps they get to see after a while that it is just as well not to say them too often to other people, too."

"Don't drive so fast, John, the day is too glorious."

Yellow butterflies flitted hither and thither down the road; the corn in the fields was turning brown and out from among it peeped here and there a pumpkin; the trees in apple orchards were bending low with their rosy and golden treasures. They passed a pool of water and saw reflected there the purple asters blooming above it. By and by the doctor turned down a grassy road leading up to a farmhouse a short distance away. "Are you to make another call today?" asked his wife.

"Yes, there is a very sick child here."

When he had gone inside three or four children came out. A curly-headed little girl edged close and looked up into Mary's face.

"Miss' Blank, *you* know where Mr. Blank got our baby, *don't* you?"

Mary, smiling down at the little questioner, said, "The doctor didn't tell me anything about it." The little faces looked surprised and disappointed.

"We thought you'd know an' we come out to ask you," said another little girl. "You make all the babies' dresses, don't you?"

"Dear me, no indeed!" laughed the doctor's wife.

"Does he keep all the babies at your house?" asked the little boy.

"I think not. I never see them there."

"Didn't he ever bring any to your house?"

"Oh, yes, five of them."

"I'd watch and see where he *gets* 'em," said the little fellow stoutly. "Jimmie Brown said Mr. Blank found their baby down in the woods in an old holler log."

The doctor came out, and the little boy looking up at him asked, "Is they any more babies down in the woods?"

"Yes, yes, 'the woods is full of 'em,'" laughed the doctor as he drove off leaving the little group quite unsatisfied.

When they had gone some distance two wagons appeared on the brow of the hill in front of them. "Hold on, Doctor," shouted the first driver, as the doctor was driving rapidly by, "I want to sell you a watermelon."

"Will you take your pay in pills?"

"Don't b'lieve I have any use for pills."

"Don't want one then, I'm broke this morning," and he passed the second wagon and pulled his horse into the road again.

"Wait a minute! *I'll* trade you a melon for some pills," called the driver. He spread the reins over the dashboard and clambered down; the man in front looked back at him with a grin. "I've got two kinds here, the Cyclone and the Monarch, which would you rather have?"

"Oh, I don't care," said the doctor.

"Let us have a Monarch, please," said Mary. Monarch was a prettier name than Cyclone, and besides there was no sense in giving so violent a name to so peaceful a thing as a watermelon. So the Monarch was brought and deposited in the back of the buggy.

The doctor opened his case. "Take your choice."

"What do you call this kind?"

"I call that kind Little Devils."

"How many of 'em would a feller dare take at once?"

"Well, I wouldn't take more than three unless you have a lawyer handy to make your will."

"Why, will they hurt me?"

"They'll bring the answer if you take enough of 'em."

The man eyed the pills dubiously,—"I believe I'll let that kind alone. What kind is this?"

"These are podophyllin pills."

"Gee, the *name's* enough to kill a feller."

"Well, Morning-Glories is a good name. If you take too many you'll be wafted straight to glory in the morning, and the road will be a little rough in places."

"Confound it, Jake," called the first driver, "don't you take *none* of 'em. Don't monkey with 'em." But Jake had agreed to trade a melon for pills. He held out his big hand. "Pour me out some of them Little Devils. I'll risk 'em."

The doctor emptied the small bottle into Jake's hand, replaced it in the case and drove off.

"John, why in the world didn't you give him some instructions as to how to take them?" asked Mary, energetically.

"He didn't ask me to prescribe for him, my dear. He wanted to trade a watermelon for pills and we traded."

"For pity's sake," said Mary indignantly, "and you're going to let that man kill himself while you strain at a point of professional etiquette!" She was gazing back at the unfortunate man.

"Don't you worry, he'll be too much afraid of them to hurt himself with them," said the doctor, laughing.

"I sincerely hope he will."

As they came in sight of home the doctor, who had been silent for some time, sighed heavily. "I am thinking of that little child out there. I tell you, Mary, a case of meningitis makes a man feel his limitations."

# CHAPTER XIII.

A long, importunate peal. The doctor rose and went swiftly. Mary listened with interest to what was to come:

"?"

"Yes."

"?"

"Yes."

"?"

"Yes."

"?"

"Yes."

"?"

"Yes."

He rang off.

"That was decided in the affirmative," said Mary.

Ting-a-ling-ling-ling. Ting-a-ling-ling-ling.

"Doctor, do you think the baby will cut any more teeth this summer?"

"You'd better ring up Solomon and ask that."

"Well—if he gets through teething—don't you think he'll be all right?"

"If he gets through with the way you *feed* him he'll be all right."

"Well, his teething has lots to do with it."

"No, it don't—not a darned bit. If you'll take care of his stomach his teeth will take care of themselves. It's what goes *between* the teeth that does the mischief. I keep telling people that every day, and once in a while I find someone with sense enough to believe it. But a lot of 'em know too much—then the baby has to pay for it."

"Well, I'll be awful careful, Doctor."

"All right then. And stick right to the baby through the hot months. Let me hear from it. Good-bye."

Ting-a-ling-ling-ling—three times. Mary rose and went. An agitated voice said, "Come and see the baby!" and was gone. "She is terribly frightened," thought Mary, as she rang central.

"Some one rang Dr. Blank. Can you find out who it was?"

"I'm afraid not."

"Will you please try?"

"Yes, but people ought to do their own talking and not bother us so much."

"I know," said Mary gently, "but this is a mother badly frightened about her baby—she did not think what she was doing and left the 'phone without giving me her name."

Central tried with such good result that Mary was soon in possession of the name and number. She telephoned that she would send the doctor down as soon as she could find him, which she thought would be in a few minutes. Then she telephoned a house where he had been for several days making evening visits.

"Is Dr. Blank there?"

"He *was* here. He's just gone."

"Is he too far away for you to call him?"

"Run and see, Tommy."

Silence. Then, "Yes, he's got too far to hear. I'm sorry."

"Very well. Thank you."

"Let me see," she meditated, "yes, I think he goes there."

She got the house. "Is Dr. Blank there?"

"He's just coming through the gate."

"Please ask him to come to the 'phone." After a minute his voice asked what was wanted and Mary delivered her message.

When her husband came home that night, she said, "John, there's one more place you're to go and you're to be there at nine o'clock."

"The deuce!" he looked at his watch, "ten minutes to nine now. Where is it?"

"I don't know."

"Don't know?"

"No. I haven't the slightest idea."

"Why didn't you find out," he asked, sharply. Mary arched her brows. "Suppose *you* find out."

John rang central. With twinkling eyes his wife listened.

"Hello, central. Who was calling Dr. Blank a while ago?"

"A good many people call, Dr. Blank. I really cannot say."

The voice was icily regular, splendidly null. It nettled the doctor.

"Suppose you try to find out."

"People who need a doctor ought to be as much interested as we are. I don't know who it was." And the receiver went up.

"Damned impudence!" said the doctor, slamming up his receiver and facing about.

"Wait, John. That girl has had to run down the woman with the sick baby. She didn't give *her* name either. Central had lots of trouble in finding her. It's small wonder she rebelled when I came at her the second time. So all I could do was to deliver the message just as it came, 'Tell the doctor to come down to our house and to be here at nine o'clock.'"

"Consultation, I suppose. They'll ring again pretty soon, I dare say, and want to know why I don't hurry up."

But nothing further was heard from the message or the messenger that night or ever after.

Ting-a-ling-ling-ling.

Can we move Henry out into the yard? It's so hot inside.

Ting-a-ling-ling-ling.

Can we move Jennie into the house? It gets pretty cold along toward morning.

Ting-a-ling-ling-ling.

Doctor, you know those pink tablets you left? I forget just how you said to take 'em.

Ting-a-ling-ling-ling.

The baby's throwing up like everything.

Ting-a-ling-ling-ling.

Johnny's swallowed a nickel!.... You say it won't?.... And not give him anything at all? Well, I needn't have been so scared, then.

Ting-a-ling-ling-ling.

The baby pulled the cat's tail and she scratched her in the face. I'm afraid she's put her eye out..... No, the *baby's* eye. I'm afraid she can't see..... No, she's not crying. She's going to sleep..... Well, I guess she *can't* see very well with her eyes shut..... Then you won't come down?.... All right, Doctor, you know best.

Ting-a-ling-ling-ling. Ting-a-ling-ling-ling.

"Is this the doctor?"

"Yes."

"The baby has a cold and I rubbed her chest with vaseline and greased her nose. Is that all right?"

"All right."

"And I am going to make her some onion syrup, if I can remember how it's made. How do you make it?"

"Why—O, *you* remember how to make it."

The truth is the doctor was not profoundly learned in some of the "home remedies" and was more helpless than the little mother herself, which she did not suspect.

"You slice the onions and put sugar on them, don't you?"

"Yes, that'll be all right," he said, hastily putting up the receiver.

Ting-a-ling-ling-ling.

"Doctor, when you come down, bring something for my fever—"

"Yes, I will!"

"And for my nervousness—"

"Yes, yes." The doctor turned quickly from the 'phone, but it rang again.

"And for my back, Doctor—"

"Yes. *Yes!*" He put the receiver up with a bang and seizing his hat rushed away before there should be any more.

Three rings.

"Is this Dr. Blank's?"

"Yes."

"Is he there?"

"No, but I expect him very soon."

"When he comes will you tell him to come out to Frank Tiller's?"

"Does he know where that is?"

"He was here once."

"Lately?"

"No, some time ago."

"Please tell me what street you live on, so the doctor will know where to go." Mary heard a consultation of a minute.

"It's on Oak street."

"East Oak or West?" Another consultation.

"North."

"Very well. I'll tell the doctor as soon as he comes."

"Tell him to come as quick as he possibly can."

Five minutes later the office ring came. Mary went obediently lest her husband might not be in. She heard the same voice ask, "Is this you, Doctor?"

"Yes."

"We want you to come out to Frank Tiller's as quick as you possibly can."

"Where is that?"

"*You've* been here."

"*Where do you live?*"

"We live on Oak street."

"East or West?"

"North."

"That street runs east and west!"

"Ma, he says the street runs east and west."

"Well, maybe it does. I've not got my directions here yet—then it must be west."

"It's on West Oak street, Doctor."

The doctor was not quite able to locate the place yet.

"Is it the house where the girl had the sore throat?"

"Ma, he says, is it the place where the girl had the sore throat?"

"It's just in front of that house."

"She says it's just in front of that house and come just as quick as you possibly can."

"What does she mean by 'in front of it'?"

"Why, it's just across the street, and come just as quick as you possibly—"

"Yes. I'll *run*."

Mary smiled, but she was glad to hear her husband add a little more pleasantly, "I'll be out there after a little."

When he came home he said, laughing, "That girl up there took the medicine I gave her and pounded the bottle to flinders before my eyes."

"What for?"

"O, she was mad."

"What did you do then?"

"Reached down in my pocket and took out another one just like it and told them to give it according to directions."

"Nothing like being prepared."

"I knew pretty well what I was up against before I went. The old complaint," said John, drawing on his slippers as he spoke.

# CHAPTER XIV.

Mary had been down the street, shopping. "I'll drop in and visit with John a few minutes," she thought, as she drew near the office. When she entered her husband was at the telephone with his back toward her.

"Hello. What is it?"

"Shake up your 'phone, I can't hear a word you're saying."

"Who?"

"Oh, yes, *I* know." Exasperation was in every letter of every word.

"Take one every six months and let me hear from you when they're all gone." Slam! "There's always *some* damned thing," he muttered, and turning faced his wife.

"A surprising prescription, John. What does it mean?"

"It means that she's one of these everlasting complainers and that I'm tired of hearing her. She's been to Chicago and St. Louis and Cincinnati. She's had three or four laparotomies and every time she comes back to me with a longer story and a worse one. They've got about everything but her appendix and they'll get that if she don't watch out."

"Why, I thought they always got that the first thing."

"You have no idea how it tires a man to have people come to him and complain, complain, *complain*. The story is ever new to them but it gets mighty old to the doctor. Then they go away to the city and some surgeon with a great name does what may seem to him to be best. Sometimes they come back improved, sometimes not, and sometimes they come back worse than when they went. In all probability the operator never sees the patient again and so the last chapters of the story must be told to the home doctor over and over again."

Mary gave a little sigh. The doctor went on:

"In many cases it isn't treatment of any kind that is needed. It is occupation—occupation for the mind and for the hands. Something that will make people forget themselves in their work or in their play."

Ting-a-ling-ling-ling. Ting-a-ling-ling-ling.

"Is this you, Doctor?"

"Yes."

"I wanted to see if you were at the office. I'll be over there right away."

In a few minutes the door opened and a gentleman about thirty-five years of age entered. His manner was greatly agitated and he did not notice Mrs. Blank at the window near the corner of the room.

"Good morning, Mr. Blake," said the doctor, shaking hands with him, "back again, are you?"

Mr. Blake had been to C—, his native city. He had not been well for some time and had evinced a desire to go back and consult his old physician there, in which Dr. Blank had heartily concurred.

"How long do you think I can live?" Mr. Blake asked now.

"What do you mean?" replied the doctor, regarding him closely.

"I want to know how much time I have. I want to get my business fixed up before—"

"Blake, you couldn't die if you wanted to. You're not a sick enough man for that."

The patient took a letter from his pocket and handed it in silence to the doctor. The latter took it, looked carefully at the superscription, read it slowly through, then folded it with cool deliberation and put it back into the envelope.

"I thought you were going to your old physician," he said.

"Dr. Kenton was out of the city so I went to the great specialist."

"Did he tell you what was in this letter he sent to me?"

"No, but the letter was not sealed and I read it. I was so anxious to know his opinion that I couldn't help it. Tuberculosis of the larynx—" his voice faltered.

"Yes," said the doctor, calmly, "that is a thing a man may well be frightened about. But listen to me, Blake. You've not got tuberculosis of the larynx."

"Do you think a great physician like Dr. Wentworth doesn't know what he is talking about?"

"Dr. Wentworth is a great physician; I know him well. But he is only a man like the rest of us and therefore liable to err in judgment sometimes. He knew you half an hour, perhaps, before he pronounced upon your case. I have known you and watched you for fifteen years. I say you have not got tuberculosis *and I know I am right.*"

Mary saw Mr. Blake grasp her husband's hand with a look in his face that made her think within herself, "Blessings on the country doctor wherever he may be, who has experience and knowledge and wisdom enough to draw just and true conclusions of his own and bravely state them when occasion demands."

When the patient had gone Mary said to her husband, "One gets a kaleidoscopic view of life in a doctor's office. What comes through the ear at home comes before the eye here. The kaleidoscope turned a bright-colored bit into the place of a dark one this time, John. I am glad I was here to see."

As she spoke footsteps were heard on the stairs. Slow and feeble steps they were, but at last they reached the landing and paused at the open door. Looking out Mary saw a poorly clad woman perhaps forty years of age, carrying in her hands a speckled hen. She was pale and trembling violently, and sank down exhausted into the chair the doctor set for her. He took the hen from her hands and set it on the floor. Its feet were securely tied and it made no effort to escape. The doctor had never seen the woman before but noting the emaciated form and the hectic flush on the cheek he saw that consumption was fast doing its work. Mary took the palm leaf fan lying on the table and stood beside her, fanning her gently.

When the woman could speak she said, "I oughtn't to 'a' tried to walk, Doctor, but there didn't seem to be anyone passin' an' this cough is killin' me. I want something for it."

"How far did you walk?" asked Mary, kindly.

"Four mile."

"Four miles!" she looked down at the trembling form with deep pity in her brown eyes.

"I didn't have any money, Doctor, but will the hen pay for the medicine?" her eyes were raised anxiously to his face and Mary's eyes met the look in the eyes of her husband.

"I don't want the hen. We haven't any place to keep her. Besides my wife, here, is afraid of hens." A little smile flitted across the wan face.

He told her how to take the medicine and then said, "Whenever you need any more let me know and I'll send it to you. You needn't worry about the pay."

"I'm very much obleeged to you, Doctor."

"Just take the hen back home with you."

"I wonder if I couldn't sell her at the store," she said, looking at the doctor with a bright, expectant face.

"Wait here and rest awhile and then we'll see about it. I'll go down and perhaps I can find some one in town from out your way that you can ride home with. Where do you live?" She told him and he went down the stairs. In a little while he came back.

"One of your neighbors is down here now waiting for you. He's just starting home," he said. He took the hen and as they started down the stairs Mary came out and joined them. At the foot of the stairway he said to the grocer standing in front of his establishment, "Here, Keller, I want you to give me a dollar for this hen."

"She ain't worth it."

"She *is* worth it," said the doctor so emphatically that Keller put his hand in his pocket and handed out the dollar. The poor woman did not see the half dollar that passed from the doctor's hand to the grocer's, but Mary saw and was glad.

The doctor laid the dollar in the trembling palm, helped the feeble woman into the wagon and they drove off.

Mary turned to her husband and said with a little break in her voice, "I'm going home, John. I want to get away from your kaleidoscope."

Ting-a-ling-ling-ling. Ting-a-ling-ling-ling.

"And I must go for another peep into it. Good-bye. Come again."

"Is this Dr. Blank?"

"Yes."

"This is Jim Sampson, Doctor, out at Sampson's mill. My boy fell out of a tree a while ago and broke his leg, and I'm sort o' worried about it."

"It don't have to *stay* broke, you know."

"That's just the point. I'm afraid it will—for a while at least."

"What do you mean?"

"Why, my wife says she won't have it set unless the signs are right for setting a broken bone. She's great on the almanac signs."

"The devil! You have that bone *set—today*! Do you understand?"

"Yes, but Mary's awful set in her way."

"I'm a darned sight more set. That boy's not going to lie there and suffer because of a fool whim of his mother's. Where is she? Send her to the 'phone and I'll talk to *her*."

"She couldn't find her almanac and ran across to the neighbor's to get one."

"Call me when she gets back."

Ten minutes passed and the call came.

"It's all right, Doctor, the signs says so."

A note of humor but of unmistakable relief vibrated in the voice.

"Come right out."

"All right, Jim, I'll be out as soon as I make my round here in town. Tell your wife to have that almanac handy. I may learn something from it."

An hour or two later he was starting out to get into the buggy, with splints and other needful things when the 'phone called him back. Hastily cramming them under the seat he went.

"Hello."

"Is this Dr. Blank?"

"This is Millie Hastings. Do you remember me?"

"No-o—I don't believe I do."

"You doctored me."

"Yes, I've 'doctored' several people."

"I had typhoid fever two years ago up in the country at my uncle's."

"What's your uncle's name?"

"Henry Peters."

"Yes, I remember now."

"I wanted to find out what my bill is."

"Wait here a moment till I look at the book."

In a minute he had found it: Millie Hastings—so many visits at such and such a date, amounting to thirty-six dollars. He went back to the 'phone.

"Do you make your money by working by the week?"

"Yes, sir."

"Have you learned how to save it?"

"Yes, sir, I had to. I have to help mother."

"Your bill is eighteen dollars."

He heard a little gasp, then a delighted voice said: "I was afraid it would be a good deal more. And now Dr. Blank, I want to ask a favor of you."

"Ask away."

"I brought four dollars to town with me today to pay on my bill, but I want a rocking chair *so* bad—I'm over here at the furniture store now—and there's such a nice one here that just costs four dollars and I thought maybe you'd wait a——"

"*Certainly* I will. Get the rocking chair by all means," and he laughed heartily as he went out to the buggy. He climbed in and drove away, the smile still lingering on his face. At the outskirts of the town a tall girl hailed him from the sidewalk. He stopped.

"I was just going to your office to get my medicine," she said.

"I left it with the man there. He'll give it to you."

"Must I take it just like the other?"

"Yes. Laugh some, though, just before you take it."

"Why?"

"Because you won't feel like it afterward."

The girl looked after him as he drove on.

"He's laughing," she said to herself and a grin overspread her face as she pursued her leisurely way.

Ting-a-ling-ling-ling-ling-ling-ling!!!

"Must be something unusual," thought Mary as the doctor went to the 'phone.

"Doctor, is this you?"

"Yes."

"Come out to John Lansing's quick!"

"What's the matter?"

"My wife swallowed poison. Hurry, Doctor, for God's sake!"

In a few minutes the doctor was on his horse (the roads being too bad for a buggy) and was off. We will follow him as he plunges along through the darkness.

Because of the mud the horse's progress was so slow that the doctor pulled him to one side, urged him on to the board walk, much against his inclination, and went clattering on at such a pace that the doors began to fly open on both sides of the street and heads, turned wonderingly after the fleeting horseman, were framed in rectangles of light.

"What *is* the matter out there?" The angle of the heads said it so plainly that the doctor laughed within himself as he thundered on. Now it chanced that one of the heads belonged to a Meddlesome Matty who, next day, stirred the matter up, and that evening two officers of the law presented themselves at Dr. Blank's office and arrested him.

"I don't care anything about the fine. All I wanted was to get there," he said, handing out the three dollars.

After the horse left the board walk the road became more solid and in about ten minutes the doctor arrived at his destination. Before he could knock the door was opened. The patient sat reclining in a chair, motionless, rigid, her eyes closed.

"What has she taken?" asked the doctor of the woman's husband.

"Laudanum."

"How much?"

"She told me she took this bottle full," and he held up a two ounce bottle.

"I think she's lying," thought the doctor as he laid his fingers upon her pulse. Then he raised the lids and looked carefully at the pupils of the eyes. "Not much contraction here," he thought. Turning to the husband who stood pale and trembling beside him, he said,

"Don't be alarmed—she's in no more danger than you are." He watched the patient's face as he spoke and saw what he expected—a faint facial movement.

"To be on the safe side we'll treat the case as if she had taken two ounces." He gave her a hypodermic emetic then called for warm water.

"How much?" asked the husband.

"O, a half gallon will do."

A big fat woman came panting through the doorway. "I got here as quick as I could," she gasped.

"We don't need you at all," said the doctor quietly. "Better go back home to your children, Mrs. Johnson."

Mrs. Johnson, not liking to be cheated out of a sensation which she dearly loved, stood still. Mr. Lansing came back with the warm water. A faint slit appeared under the eyelids of the patient. The doctor took the big cup and said abruptly, "Here! drink this!"

No response. "Mrs. Lansing!" he said so sharply that her eyes opened. "Drink this water."

"I ca-an't," she murmured feebly.

"Yes, you can."

"I won't," the voice was getting stronger.

"You will."

"You'll see."

"Yes, I'll see."

He held the big vessel to her mouth. When the water began to pour down her neck she sprang to her feet fighting it off. He held the cup in his left hand while with his right he reached around her neck and took her firmly by the nose. Then he held the cup against her mouth and when it opened for breath he poured the life-saving fluid forcefully down. Great gulps of it were swallowed while a wide sheet of water poured down her neck and over her night-dress to the floor.

"That was very well done. Better sit down now."

The husband stood in awed silence. The fat woman shook her fist at the doctor's back which he beheld, nothing daunted, in the looking-glass on the wall. The patient herself sat down in absolute quiet. In a minute she began retching and vomited some of the water. The doctor inspected it carefully. Then he went to his overcoat on a chair, felt in the pocket and drew out a coil of something. It looked like red rubber and was about half an inch in diameter. He slowly unwound it. It was five or six feet in length. A subdued voice asked,

"What are you going to do now, Doctor?"

"I am going to turn on the hose."

"Wha-a-t?"

"I am going to put this tube down into your stomach. You haven't thrown up much of that laudanum yet."

She opened her mouth to speak and the doctor inserted one end of the tube and began ramming it down. "Unfasten a button or two here," he said to her husband and rammed some more. She gagged and gurgled and tried to push his hands away.

"Hold on, we're not down yet—we're only about to the third button." He began ramming the tube again when she looked up at her husband so imploringly that he said, "Hold on a minute, Doctor, she wants to say something." The doctor withdrew the tube and waited.

"I'm sure I threw it all up."

"Oh no," he said beginning to lift it again.

"I—only—took—two—or three drops."

"Why the devil didn't you say so at the start?"

"I wish I had. I just told *Jim* that."

"To get even with him for something," announced the doctor quietly.

"How can he know so much," mused Jim's wife.

"Now I advise you not to try this game again," said the doctor as he wound up the stomach tube and put it into his pocket. "You can't fool Jim all the time, and you can't fool me any of the time. Good night." And he rode home and found Mary asleep in her chair.

Ting-a-ling-ling-ling. Ting-a-ling-ling-ling.

"Is this you, Dr. Blank?"

"Yes."

"I wanted to ask you about an electric vibrator."

"About what?"

"An electric vibrator."

"An electric something—I didn't get the last word."

A little laugh, then "v-i-b-r-a-t-o-r."

"Oh! vibrator."

"Yes. Do you think it would help my aunt?"

"Not a durned bit."

Another little laugh, "You don't think it would?"

"No!"

"I had a letter today from my cousin and she said she knew a lady who had had a stroke and this vibrator helped her more than anything."

"It didn't. She imagined it."

"Well, I didn't know anything about it and I knew you would, so I thought I'd 'phone you before going any further. Much obliged, Doctor."

It would save much time and money and disappointment if all those who don't know would pause to put a question or two to those who do. But so it is *not*, and the maker of worthless devices and the concocter of nostrums galore cometh oft to fortune by leaps and bounds, while the poor, conscientious physician who sticks to the truth of things, arriveth betimes at starvation's gate.

(I was startled a few days ago to learn that the average income of physicians in the United States does not exceed six hundred dollars.)

Ting-a-ling-ling-ling. Ting-a-ling-ling-ling.

"Tell papa he's wanted at the 'phone," said Mary.

"Where is he?"

"Isn't he there in the dining room?"

"No, he isn't here."

"He must be in the kitchen then; go to the door and call him."

The small boy obeyed. "He's not out here either," he announced from the door-way.

"Why, where can he be!" cried Mary, springing up and going swiftly to the 'phone. "Hello."

"Is the doctor there?"

"Yes. Wait just a minute and I will call him."

She hurried through the dining room, then through the kitchen and out into the yard. No doctor to be seen. "He passed through the house not three minutes ago," she said to herself.

"John!"

"Doctor!"

"Doc-*tor*!"

"O, dear! I don't see how he could disappear from the face of the earth in three minutes' time!"

She hurried around a projecting corner through a little gate and called again.

"What is it?" asked a placid voice as its owner emerged from his new auto garage.

"Hurry to the 'phone for pity's sake!" and he hurried. Mary, following, all out of breath, heard this:

"Two teaspoonfuls." Then the doctor hung up the receiver. He turned to Mary and laughed as he quoted Emerson on the mountain and the mouse.

"I chased you all over the place this afternoon, John, when the 'phone was calling you, and couldn't find you at all. Some people have days to 'appear' but this seems to be your day to disappear. Where were you then?"

"Out in the garage."

"Fascinating spot! I'll know where to look next time. Now come to supper."

# CHAPTER XV.

It was October—the carnival time of the year,

When on the ground red apples lie

In piles like jewels shining,

And redder still on old stone walls

Are leaves of woodbine twining.

When comrades seek sweet country haunts,

By twos and twos together,

And count like misers, hour by hour,

October's bright blue weather.

On a lovely afternoon our travelers were driving leisurely along through partially cleared woodland. The doctor had proposed that they take this trip in the new automobile. But Mary had declined with great firmness.

"I will not be hurled along the road in October of all months. What fools these mortals be," she went on. "Last year while driving slowly through the glorious Austrian Tyrol fairly holding my breath with delight, one machine after another whizzed by, the occupants fancying they were 'doing' the Tyrol, I dare say."

Mary looked about her, drinking in deep draughts of the delicious air. The beautifully-tinted leaves upon every tree and bush, the blue haze in the distance and the dreamful melancholy over all, were delightful to her. The fragrance of wild grapes came to them as they emerged from the woods and Mary said, "Couldn't you wait a minute, John, until I go back and find them? I'll bring you some."

"If you were sick and had sent for a doctor would you like to have him fool around gathering grapes and everything else on his way?"

"No, I wouldn't. I really wouldn't."

They laughed as they sped along the open country road, skirted on either side by a rail fence. From a fence corner here and there arose tall sumac, like candelabra bearing aloft their burning tapers. The poke-weed flung out its royal purple banners while golden-rod and asters were blooming everywhere. Suddenly Mary exclaimed, "I'm going to get out of the buggy this minute."

"What for?"

"To gather those brown bunches of hazelnuts."

"Mary, I positively will not wait for you."

"John, I positively don't want you to wait for me," said Mary, putting her foot on the step, "I'm going to stay here and gather nuts till you come back. See how many there are?" and she sprang lightly to the ground.

"It will be an hour or more before I can get back. I've got to take up that pesky artery."

"It won't seem long. You know I like to be alone."

"Good-bye, then," and the doctor started off.

"Wait! John," his wife called after him. "I haven't a thing to put the nuts in, please throw me the laprobe." The doctor crushed the robe into a sort of bundle and threw it to her.

She spread the robe upon the ground and began plucking the bunches. Her fingers flew nimbly over the bushes and soon she had a pile of the brown treasures. Dear old times came trooping back. She thought of far-off autumn days when she had taken her little wagon and gone out to the hazel bushes growing near her father's house, and filled it to the top and tramped it down and filled it yet again. Then a gray October day came back when three or four girls and boys, all busy in the bushes, talked in awed tones of the great fire—Chicago was burning up! Big, big Chicago, which they had never seen or dreamed of seeing—all because a cow kicked over a lamp.

Mary moved to another clump of bushes. As she worked she thought if she had never known the joy of gathering nuts and wild grapes and persimmons, of wandering through woods and meadows, her childhood would have lost much that is beautiful and best, and her womanhood many of its dearest recollections.

"You're the doctor's wife, ain't ye?"

Mary looked around quite startled. A tall woman in a blue calico dress and a brown gingham sunbonnet was standing there. "I didn't want to scare ye, I guess you didn't see me comin'."

"I didn't know you were coming—yes, I am the doctor's wife."

"We saw ye from the house and supposed he'd gone on to see old man Benning and that you had stopped to pick nuts."

"You guessed it exactly," said Mary with a smile.

"We live about a quarter mile back from the road so I didn't see the doctor in time to stop him."

"Is some one sick at your house, then?"

"Well, my man ain't a doin' right, somehow. He's been ailin' for some time and his left foot and leg is a turnin' blue. I come to see if you could tell me somethin' I could do for it. I'm afraid it's mortifyin'."

Mary's brown eyes opened wide. "Why, my dear woman, I couldn't tell you anything to do. I don't know anything at all about such things."

"I supposed bein' a doctor's wife you'd learnt everything like that."

"I have learned many things by being a doctor's wife, very many things, but what to do with a leg and foot that are mortifying I really could not tell you." Mary turned her face away to hide a laugh that was getting near the surface. "I will have the doctor drive up to the house when he gets back if you wish," she said, turning to her companion.

"Maybe that would be best. Your husband cured me once when I thought nothing would ever get me well again. I think more of him than any other man in the world."

"Thank you. So do I."

She started off and Mary went on gathering nuts, her face breaking into smiles at the queer errand and the restorative power imputed to herself. "If it is as serious as she thinks, all the doctors in the world can't do much for it, much less one meek and humble doctor's wife. But they could amputate, I suppose, and I'm sure I couldn't, not in a scientific way."

Thus soliloquizing, she went from clump to clump of the low bushes till they were bereft of their fruitage. She looked down well-pleased at the robe with the nuts piled upon it. She drew the corners up and tied her bundle securely. This done she looked down the road where the doctor had disappeared. "I'll just walk on and meet him," she thought. She went leisurely along, stopping now and then to pluck a spray of goldenrod. When she had gathered quite a bunch she looked at it closely. "You are like some people in this world—you have a pretty name and at a little distance *you* are pretty: but seen too close you are a disappointment, and more than that you are coarse. I don't want you," and she flung them away. She saw dust rising far down the road and hoped it might be the doctor. Yes, it was he, and Bucephalus seemed to know that he was traveling toward home. When her husband came up and she was seated beside him, she said, "You are wanted at that little house over yonder," and she told him what had taken place in the hazel bushes. "You're second choice though, they came for me first," she said laughing.

"I wish to thunder you'd gone. They owe me a lot now they'll never pay."

"At any rate, they hold you in very high esteem, John."

"Oh, yes, but esteem butters no bread."

"Well, you'll go, won't you? I told the woman you would."

"Yes, I'll go."

He turned into a narrow lane and in a few minutes they were at the gate. The doctor handed the reins to Mary and went inside. A girl fourteen or fifteen years old with a bald-headed baby on her arm came out of the house and down the path.

"Won't you come in?"

"No, thank you. We will be going home in a minute."

The girl set the baby on the gate-post. "She's the smartest baby I ever saw," she said. "She's got a whole mouthful of teeth already."

"And how old is she?"

"She was ten months old three weeks ago last Saturday."

As today was Thursday, Mary was on the point of saying, "She will be eleven months old in a few days then," but checked herself—she understood. It would detract from the baby's smartness to give her eleven months instead of only ten in which to accomplish such wonders in the way of teeth. The doctor came out and they started. Just before they came out to the main road they passed an old deserted house. No signs of life were about it except the very luxuriant life in the tall jimsons and ragweeds growing about it and reaching almost to the top of the low doorway, yawning blackly behind them.

"I think the longest night of my life was spent in that house about sixteen years ago. It's the only house I was ever in where there was nothing at all to read. There wasn't even an almanac."

Mary laughed. "An almanac is a great deal better than nothing, my dear. I found that out once upon a time when I had to stay in a house for several hours where there was just one almanac and not another printed page. I read the jokes two or three times till they began to pall and then set to work on the signs. I'll always have a regard for them because they gave me a lift through those tedious hours."

They were not far from the western edge of the piece of woodland they were traversing and all about them was the soft red light of the setting sun. They could see the sun himself away off through the straight and solemn trunks of the trees. A mile farther on Mary uttered a sudden exclamation of delight.

"See that lovely bittersweet!"

"I see, but don't ask me to stop and get you some."

"I won't, but I'll ask you to stop and let *me* get some."

"I wouldn't bother about it. You'll have to scramble over that ditch and up the bank—"

"I've scrambled over worse things in my life," she said, springing from the buggy and picking her way down the intervening ditch. The bright red berries in their flaring yellow hoods were beautiful. She began breaking off the branches. When she had gathered a large bunch and was turning toward the buggy she saw a vehicle containing two women approaching from the opposite direction. There was a ditch on either side of the road which, being narrow at this point, made passing a delicate piece of work. The doctor drew his horse to one side so that the wheels of the buggy rested on the very brink and waited for them to pass; he saw that there was room with perhaps a foot or two to spare.

On came the travelers and—the front wheels of the two vehicles were locked in a close embrace. For a minute the doctor did some vigorous thinking and then he climbed out of the buggy. It was a trying position. He could not say all of the things he wanted to—it would not be polite; neither did he want to act as if it were nothing because Mary might not understand the extent of the mischief she had caused and how much out of humor he was with her. It would be easier if she were only out of hearing instead of looking at him across the ditch with apologetic eyes.

The doctor's horse began to move uneasily but the other stood perfectly still.

"He's used to this sort of thing, perhaps," said the doctor with as little sarcasm as possible.

"Yes, we have run into a good many buggies and things," said one of the women, cheerfully.

"Women beat the devil when it comes to driving," thought the doctor within himself. "They'll drive right over you and never seem to think they ought to give part of the road. And they do it everywhere, not only where there are ditches." He restrained his speech, backed the offending vehicle and started the travelers on. While he was doing so his own steed started on and he had a lively run to catch him.

Mary had thought of turning back to break off another spray of the bittersweet but John's profanity was rising to heaven. Diplomacy required her to get to the buggy and into it at once. This she did and the doctor plunged in after her.

"Forgive me for keeping you waiting," she said gently. She held the bittersweet out before her. "Isn't it lovely, John?"

A soft observation turneth away wrath. The doctor's was oozing away sooner than he wished.

They drove on for a while in silence. The soft, still landscape dotted here and there with farm houses and with graceful elm and willow trees, was lit up and glorified by the after-glow. The evening sky arching serenely over a quiet world, how beautiful it was! And as Mary's eyes caught a glittering point of light in the blue vault above them, she sang softly to herself:

"O, thou sublime, sweet evening star,

Joyful I greet thee from afar."

For a while she watched the stars as one by one they twinkled into view, then drawing her wraps more closely about her, she leaned back in the carriage and gave herself up to pleasant reflection, and before she realized it the lights of home were twinkling cheerily ahead.

# CHAPTER XVI.

"You are not going out tonight, John, no matter how often the 'phone rings. I positively will not let you." Mary spoke with strong emphasis. All the night before he had been up and today had been a hard day for him. She had seldom seen him so utterly weary as he was tonight. He had come home earlier than usual and now sat before the fire, his head sunk on his breast, half asleep.

"Go right to bed, dear, then you can really rest."

The doctor, too tired to offer any resistance, rose and went to the bedroom. In a few minutes his wife heard regular sonorous sounds from the bed. (When she spoke of these sounds to John, Mary pronounced it without the first *o*.)

Glad that he had so soon fallen into deep sleep she settled back in her chair. "I'll protect him tonight," she thought, "though fiery darts be hurled."

She thought of many things. The fire-light gleamed red upon the hearth. All was still. The sounds from the adjoining room had ceased. Something stirred within her and she rose and went softly to the bedside of her sleeping husband. In the half-light she could see the strong, good face. Dear John so profane yet so patient, so severe yet so tender, what would it be to face life without him. She laid her hand very lightly on the hand which lay on the counterpane, then took it away lest it disturb the sleeper. She went back to her chair and opening a little volume took from it a folded sheet. Twice before today had she read the words written within it. A dear friend whose husband had recently died had written her, inclosing them. She read them again now:

## IN MEMORIAM,—A PRAYER.

"O God! The Father of the spirits of all flesh, in whatsoever world or condition they be,—I beseech Thee for him whose name, and dwelling place, and every need Thou knowest. Lord, vouchsafe him peace and light, rest and refreshment, joy and consolation in Paradise, in the ample folds of Thy great love. Grant that his life, so troubled here, may unfold itself in Thy sight, and find employment in the spacious fields of Eternity.—If he hath ever been hurt or maimed by any unhappy word or deed of mine, I pray Thee, of Thy great pity, to heal and restore him, that he may serve Thee without hindrance.

"Tell him, O gracious Father, if it may be,—how much I love him and miss him, and long to see him again; and if there may be ways in which he may come, vouchsafe him to me as guide and guard, and grant me such sense of his nearness as Thy laws permit. If in aught I can minister to his peace, be pleased of Thy love to let this be; and mercifully keep me from every act which may deprive me of the sight of him, as soon as our trial time is over, or mar the fullness of our joy when the end of the days hath come."

Mary brushed away a tear from her cheek. "This letter has awakened unusual thoughts. I will—"

A sharp peal from the telephone.

"What is it?"

"Is the doctor at home?"

"Yes. He has gone to bed and is fast asleep."

"Oh! We wanted him to come down to see my sister."

"He was up all last night and is not able to come—"

"Can I just talk to him about her?"

Mary sighed. To rouse him from his sorely needed sleep was too cruel. Then she spoke. "I must not disturb him unless it is absolutely necessary. I shall be sitting here awake—call me again in a little while if you think it necessary."

"A—l—l r—i—g—h—t—" and a sob came distinctly to the listener's ear.

This was too much for Mary. "I'll call him," she said hurriedly and went to the bedroom.

With much difficulty she roused him. He threw back the covers, got up and stumbled to the 'phone.

"Hello..... Yes..... They didn't? Is she suffering much?.... All right, I'll be down in a little bit."

Mary groaned aloud. She had vowed to protect him though fiery darts be hurled. But the sob in the voice of a frightened young girl was more potent than any fiery dart could have been and had melted her at once. Slowly but surely the doctor got himself into his clothes.

"I don't think there's any use of my going down there again, but I suppose I'll have it to do." When he returned an hour later, he said, "Just as I thought—they were badly scared over nothing. I shouldn't wonder if they'd rout me out again before morning."

"No, they won't," said Mary to herself, and when her husband was safe in bed again, she walked quietly to the telephone, took down the receiver and *left* it down. "Extreme cases require extreme measures," she thought as she, too, prepared for her night's rest. But there was a haunting feeling in her mind about the receiver hanging there. Suppose some one who really did need the doctor should call and call in vain. She would not think of it. She turned over and fell asleep and they both slept till morning and rose refreshed for another day.

A few weeks later circumstances much like those narrated above arose, and the doctor's wife for the second and last time left the receiver down. About two o'clock there came a tragic pounding at the door and when the doctor went to open it a voice asked, "What's the matter down here?"

"Why?"

"Central's been ringing you to beat the band and couldn't get you awake."

"Strange we didn't hear. What's wanted?" He had recognized the messenger as the night clerk at the hotel not far from his home.

"A man hurt at the railroad—they're afraid he'll bleed to death. Central called me and asked me to run over here and rouse you."

When the doctor was gone Mary rose tremblingly and hung up the receiver. She would not tell John what she had done. He would be angry. She had felt that the end justified the means—that he was tired out and half sick and sorely needed a night's unbroken rest—but if the end should be the bleeding to death of this poor man—

She dared not think of it. She went back to bed but not to sleep. She lay wide awake keenly anxious for her husband's return. And when at last he came her lips could hardly frame the question, "How is he, John?"

"Pretty badly hurt, but not fatally."

"Thank heaven!" Mary whispered, and formed a quick resolve which she never broke. This belonged to her husband's life—it must remain a part of it to the end.

# CHAPTER XVII.

One lovely morning in April, Mary was called to the telephone.

"I want you to drive to the country with me this morning," said her husband.

"I'll be delighted. I have a little errand down town and I'll come to the office—we can start from there." Accordingly half an hour later she walked into the office and seated herself in a big chair to wait till John was ready. The door opened and a small freckle-faced boy entered.

"Good morning, Governor," said the doctor. The governor grinned.

"What can I do for you today?"

"How much will ye charge to pull a tooth?"

"Well, I'll pull the tooth and if it don't hurt I won't charge anything. Sit down."

The boy sat down and the doctor got out his forceps. The tooth came hard but he got it. The boy clapped his hand over his mouth but not a sound escaped him.

"There it is," said the doctor, holding out the offending member. "Do you want it?" A boy's tooth is a treasure to be exhibited to all one's friends. He took it and put it securely in his pocket.

"How much do I have to pay?"

"Did it hurt?"

"Nope."

"Nothing at all."

The boy slid from the chair and out of the door, ecstasy overspreading all the freckles.

"That boy has a future," said Mary looking after him with a smile.

"I see they have brought the horse. We must be starting."

Ting-a-ling-ling-ling. Ting-a-ling-ling-ling.

"They want ye down at Pete Jansen's agin."

"What's the matter there now?"

"O, that youngun's been *drinkin'* somethin' agin."

"Into the lye this time, too?"

"No, it's coal oil and bluin' this time and I don't know what else."

"I'll be down right away," said the doctor, taking up his hat.

"Get into the buggy and drive down with me, Mary, it's just at the edge of town and then we can drive on into the country."

When they stopped at the house, an unpainted little frame structure, Mary held the horse while her husband went in.

"Where's the boy?" he asked, looking around.

"He's out in the back yard a-playin' now, I guess," his mother replied from the bed.

"Then what in thunder did you send for me for?"

"Why, I was scared for fear it would kill him." The doctor turned to go then paused to ask, "How's the baby?"

"She's doin' fine."

"She's just about a week old now, isn't she?"

"A week yesterday. Don't you want to see how much she's growed?"

The doctor went to the bed and looked down at the wee little maiden.

"Great God!" he exclaimed, so fiercely that the woman was frightened. "Why haven't you let me know about this baby's eyes?"

"W'y, we didn't think it'd 'mount to anything. We thought they'd git well in a day or two."

"She'll be blind in less than a week if something isn't done for them."

"Grandmother's been a doctorin' 'em some."

"Well, there's going to be a change of doctors right straight. I'm going to treat this baby's eyes myself."

"We don't want any strong medicine put in a baby's eyes."

"It don't make a bit of difference what you want. I'm going to the drug store now to get what I need and I want you to have warm water and clean cloths ready by the time I get back. Is there anyone here to do it?"

"There's a piece of a girl out there in the kitchen. She ain't much 'count." The doctor went to the kitchen door and gave his orders.

"I'd ruther you'd let the baby's eyes alone. I'm afraid to have strong medicine put in 'em."

For answer he went out, got into the buggy and drove rapidly back to town where he procured what he needed and in a few minutes was back.

"You'd better come in this time, Mary, you'll get tired of waiting and besides I want you to see this baby. I want you to know something about what every father and mother ought to understand."

They went in and the doctor took the baby up and seated himself by the chair on which stood a basin of water. The mother, with very ungracious demeanor, looked on. Mary, shocked and filled with pity, looked down into the baby's face. The inflammation in the eyes was terrible. The secretion constantly exuded and hung in great globules to the tiny lids. Never in her life had she seen anything like it. "Let me hold it for you," she said, sitting down and taking the baby in her lap.

The doctor turned the little head toward him and held it gently between his knees. He took a pair of goggles from his pocket and put them over his eyes to protect them from the poison, then tenderly as any mother could have done, he bathed and cleansed the poor little eyes opening so inauspiciously upon the world. He thought as he worked of this terrible scourge of infancy, producing one-third of all the blindness in the world. He thought too, that almost all of this blindness was preventable by prompt and proper treatment. Statistics had proven these two things beyond all doubt. He thought of the earnest physicians who had labored long to have some laws enacted in regard to this stupendous evil but with little result.[1]

[1] 1. Ophthalmia Neonatorum

2. There has been legislation for the prevention of blindness in the States of New York, Maine, Rhode Island and Illinois.

When they were in the buggy again Mary said, "But what if the baby goes blind after all? Of course they would say that you did it with your 'strong medicine.'"

"Of course they would, but that would not disturb me in the least. But it will not go blind now. I'll see to that."

Soon they had left the town behind them and were fairly on their way. The soft, yet bracing, air of the April morning was delightful. The sun shone warm. Birds carolled everywhere. The buds on the oak trees were swelling, while those on the maples were bursting into red and furzy bloom. Far off to the left a tall sycamore held out white arms in welcome to the Springtime and perfect stillness lay upon the landscape.

"I am so glad the long reign of winter and bad roads is ended, John, so I can get out with you again into the blessed country."

"And I am glad to have good company."

"Thanks for that gallant little speech. Ask me often, but I won't go every time because you might get tired of me and I'd be sure to get tired of you."

"Thanks for that gracious little speech."

That evening when the doctor and Mary were sitting alone, she said, "John, that baby's eyes have haunted me all day long. And you say one-third of the blindness of the world is due to this disease."

"Yes."

"That seems to me a terrific accusation against you doctors. What have you been doing to prevent it?"

"Everything that has been done—not very much, I'm afraid. Speaking for myself, I can say that I have long been deeply interested. I have written several papers on the subject—one for our State Medical Society."

"So far so good. But I'd like to know more about it."

"Write to the secretary of the State Board of Health for all the information that he can give you."

The next day Mary wrote. Three days later she received the following letter:

Springfield, Nov. 16, 1909.

My dear Mrs. Blank:

Several states of the Union have laws in relation to the prevention of blindness, some good, some bad, and some indifferent, and I fear that the last applies to the manner in which the laws are enforced in the majority of the States. In the December, 1908, *Bulletin* of this Board, a copy of which I send you under separate cover, you will find the Illinois law, which, as you can readily see, is very difficult of enforcement.

But, as I said, much can be done in its enforcement if the State Board of Health can secure the co-operation of the physicians of the State. However, in this connection you will note that I have made an appeal to physicians, on page 757. Yet, to the best of my knowledge, the Board has not received one inquiry in regard to the enforcement of this law, except from the Committee on the Prevention of Ophthalmia Neonatorum.

In regard to the other States, it will take me some time to look up the laws, but I will advise you in a few days.

Sincerely yours,

J. A. Egan.

After reading it carefully through, Mary's eye went back to the sentence, "Much can be done if the State Board of Health can secure the co-operation of the physicians of the State."

She rose and walked the floor. "If I were a Voice—a persuasive voice," she thought, "I would fly to the office of every physician in our great State and then to every physician in the land and would whisper in his ear, 'It is your glorious privilege to give light to sightless eyes. It is more: it is your sacred duty. O, be up and doing!'"

"To think, John," she said, turning impetuously toward her husband, "that I, all these years the wife of a man who knows this terrible truth, should just be finding it out. Then think of the thousands of men and women who know nothing about it. How are they to know? Who is to tell them? Who is to blame for the blindness in the first place? Who can—"

Ting-a-ling-ling-ling. Ting-a-ling-ling-ling. Ting-a-ling-ling-ling.

"Is this Dr. Blank?"

"Yes."

"This is Mr. Ardmore. Can you come up to my house right away?"

"Right away."

When he arrived at his destination he was met at the door by a well-dressed, handsome young man. "Just come into this room for a few minutes, Doctor. My wife says they are not quite ready for you in there."

"Who is the patient?" asked the doctor as he walked into the room indicated.

"The baby boy."

"The baby boy!" exclaimed the doctor. "I didn't know the little rascal had got here."

"Yes, you were out of town. My wife and I thought that ended the matter but he got here just the same."

"Mighty glad to hear it. How old is he?"

"Just ten days."

"Pretty fine, isn't he?"

"You bet! I wouldn't take all the farms in these United States for him."

"To be sure. To be sure," laughed the doctor. He picked up a little volume lying open on the table. "Do you like Omar?" he asked, aimlessly turning the pages.

"Very much. I don't always get the old Persian's meaning exactly. Take this verse," he reached for the book and turning back a few pages read:

"The moving finger writes; and having writ,

Moves on; nor all your piety nor wit

Shall lure it back to cancel half a line,

Nor all your tears wash out a word of it.

That sounds pretty but it has something in it that almost scares a fellow— he doesn't know why."

The nurse appeared in the doorway and announced that the doctor might come in now. Both men rose and went across the hall into the bedroom. The doctor shook hands with the baby's mother. "Where did you get this?" he asked, laying his hand on the downy little head.

"He came out of the everywhere into the here," she quoted, smiling.

"Nurse, turn the baby's face up so the doctor can see his eyes. They're greatly inflamed, Doctor," she said.

The doctor started. "Bring a light closer," he said sharply.

While the light was being brought he asked, "Did this inflammation begin when the baby was about three days old?"

"He was exactly three days old."

"And been growing worse ever since?"

"Yes. Dr. Brown was with me when he was born. He came in the next day and everything was all right. Then he was called to Chicago and I didn't know enough about babies to know that this might be serious."

"*You* ought to have known," said the doctor sternly, turning to the nurse.

"I am not a professional nurse. I have never seen anything like this before."

The light was brought and the nurse took the baby in her arms. The doctor, bending over it, lifted the swollen little lids and earnestly scrutinized the eyes. *The cornea was entirely destroyed!*

"O God!" The words came near escaping him. Sick at heart he turned his face away that the mother might not see. She must not know the awful truth until she was stronger. He gave some instructions to the nurse, then left the room followed by the baby's father.

"Stop for a few minutes, Doctor, if you please. I'd like to ask you something about this," and both resumed their seats, after Mr. Ardmore had closed the door.

"Do you think the baby's eyes have been hurt by too much light?"

"No by darkness—Egyptian darkness."

The young man looked at him in wonder.

"What is the disease?"

"It is Ophthalmia Neonatorum, or infantile sore eyes."

"What is the nature of it?"

"It is always an infection."

"How can that be? There has been nobody at all in the room except Dr. Brown and the nurse."

The doctor did not speak. There came into his mind the image of Mary as she had asked so earnestly, "How are they to know? Who is to tell them?"

Leaning slightly forward and looking the young man in the face he said, "I do not know absolutely, but *you* know!"

"Know what?"

"Whether or not your child's eyes have had a chance to be infected by certain germs."

"What do you mean, Doctor?" asked the young father in vague alarm.

Slowly, deliberately, and with keen eyes searching the other's face the doctor made reply:

"I mean that the sins of the fathers are visited upon the children."

There was bewildered silence for an instant then a wave of crimson surged over neck, cheek and brow. It was impossible to meet the doctor's eyes. The young man looked down and made no attempt to speak. By and by he said in a low voice, "It's no use for me to deny to you, Doctor, that I have been a fool and have let my base passions master me. But if I had dreamed of any such result as this they wouldn't have mastered me—I know that."

"The man that scorns these vile things because of the eternal wrong in them will never have any fearful results rising up to confront him."

"All that has been put behind me forever, Doctor; I feel the truth and wisdom of what you say. Just get my boy's eyes well and he shall never be ashamed of his father."

The doctor looked away from the handsome, intelligent face so full at that moment of love and tenderness for this new son which had been given into his care and keeping, and a wave of pity surged over him. But he must go on to the bitter end.

"You have not understood this old Persian's verse," he said, taking up the little book again. "Tonight his meaning is to be made plain to you."

Slowly he read:

"The Moving Finger writes; and, having writ,

Moves on; nor all your Piety nor Wit

Shall lure it back to cancel half a Line,

Nor all your Tears wash out a Word of it."

He laid the volume gently down and turning, faced the younger man.

"Listen: In those licentious days the Moving Finger was writing a word for the future to reveal. It wrote BLIND in the eyes of your helpless child."

"My God! You don't mean it!"

"It is true. The cornea is destroyed."

A deathly pallor overspread the young man's face. He bowed his head in his hands and great sobs shook his frame. "My God! My God!" he gasped over and over again. Accustomed as the doctor was to suffering and sorrow this man's anguish was too much for him. The tears rolled down his cheeks and he made no effort to restrain them.

After a long time the younger man raised his head and spoke in broken words, "Doctor, I must not keep you here. You are needed elsewhere. Leave me to Remorse. I am young and you are growing old, Doctor, but will you take this word from me? You and all in your profession should long ago have told us these things. The world should not lie in ignorance of this tremendous evil. If men will not be saved from themselves they will save their unborn children, if they only know. God help them."

The doctor went slowly homeward, his mind filled with the awful calamity in the household he had left. "It is time the world is waking," he thought. "We must arouse it."

Ting-a-ling-ling-ling. Ting-a-ling-ling-ling. Ting-a-ling-ling-ling.

"Is this Mrs. Blank?"

It was a manly voice vibrating with youth and joy.

"I want to tell you that your husband has just left a sweet little daughter at our house."

"Oh, has he! I'm very glad, Mr. Farwell. Thank you for telephoning. Father, mother and baby all doing well?"

"Fine as silk. I had to tell *somebody* right away. Now I'm off to send some telegrams to the folks at home. Goodbye."

Ting-a-ling-ling-ling. Ting-a-ling-ling-ling. Ting-a-ling-ling-ling.

"This is Mrs. Blank is it not?"

"Yes."

"Will you please tell the doctor that father is dead. He died twenty minutes ago."

"The doctor was expecting the message, Mr. Jameson," said Mary gently. This, too, was the voice of a young man, but quiet, subdued, bringing tidings of death instead of life. And Mary, going back to her seat in the twilight, thought of the words of one—Life is a narrow vale between the cold and barren peaks of two eternities. The eternity before the baby came, the eternity after the old man went, were solemnly in her thoughts. But they were not cold and barren peaks to her. They were crowned with light and warmth and love.

And into her thoughts came, too, the never-ending story of the 'phone as it was unfolding itself to her throughout the years. Humor and pathos, folly and wisdom, tragedy and comedy, pain, anguish, love, joy, sorrow—all had spoken and had poured their brief story into the listening ear of the helper. And when he was not there, into the ear of one who must help in her own poor way.

O countless, countless messages stored in her memory to await his coming! Only she could know how faithfully she had guarded and delivered them. Only she could—

Ting-a-ling. Ting-a-ling. Ting-a-ling-ling-ling.

Milton Keynes UK
Ingram Content Group UK Ltd.
UKHW020828231024
450026UK00004B/451